Current Practice in
Health Sciences Librarianship

Alison Bunting

Editor-in-Chief

Volume 8
Administration and Management in
Health Sciences Libraries

Edited by
Rick B. Forsman

Medical Library Association
and
The Scarecrow Press, Inc.
Lanham, Maryland, and London

British Library Cataloguing-in-Publication Information Available

Library of Congress Cataloging-in-Publication Data

Administration and management in health sciences libraries / edited by Rick B. Forsman
    p. cm.—(Current practice in health sciences librarianship ; v. 8)
    Includes bibliographical references and index.
    ISBN 0-8108-3896-6 (acid-free paper)
        1. Medical libraries—United States—Administration. I. Forsman, Rick B. II. Series.

    Z675.M4 A36 2000   00-056082
    026.61—dc21

Printed on acid-free paper

♾™ The paper used in this publication meets the minimum requirements of
American National Standard for Information Sciences—Permanence of Paper
for Printed Library Materials, ANSI/NISO Z39.48-1992.

Administration and Management in Health Sciences Libraries

Contents

Preface / *Alison Bunting*   vii

Expert Reviewers   xi

Advisory Committee Members   xiii

Authors   xv

Introduction / *Rick B. Forsman*   xvii

1   Management Challenges in an Era of Change: An Overview / *Barbara A. Epstein, Patricia C. Mickelson, and Ellen G. Detlefsen*   1

2   Fiscal Management in Health Sciences Libraries / *Lynn Kasner Morgan*   19

3   Human Resources Management / *Carol Jenkins*   35

4   Marketing Library Services / *Joan S. Ash and Elizabeth H. Wood*   75

5   The Technological Transformation of Health Sciences Libraries / *Audrey Powderly Newcomer*   101

6   Planning for Health Sciences Library Facilities / *Frieda O. Weise and Mary Joan (M.J.) Tooey*   133

7   The Application of Systematic Research / *Prudence W. Dalrymple*   173

Appendix A: Compilation of Skills Recommended for Careers in Health Sciences Librarianship   195

Appendix B: Annotated Bibliography of Library Space Planning   199

Glossary   205

Index   209

Author Biographies   219

Preface

Current Practice in Health Sciences Librarianship (CPHSL) continues the publication principles established by its predecessor, the *Handbook of Medical Library Practice:* to serve as a general introduction to the field of health sciences librarianship for graduate students; a source of basic information and references to the literature for the Medical Library Association's (MLA) professional development and recognition program; a reference work for health sciences librarians and other information specialists, providing basic information in areas peripheral to their own expertise; and a means of documenting the state of practice of health sciences librarianship at a particular point in time.

The decision to change the title of this venerable MLA publication is best explained by a review of the *Handbook's* publication history. The appearance in 1942 of the first edition of the *Handbook*, published by the American Library Association, fulfilled a long-standing goal of the MLA. As editor Janet Doe noted:

> The demand [for a handbook] has grown keener with the passage of time, undoubtedly because of the recent rapid increase in the number of medical libraries, for half of the 315 now existing in this country have originated since 1910. To staff these libraries, workers have been enticed or commandeered from general and special libraries, from library schools, from the clerical staff of hospitals or medical schools, and from doctors' offices [1].

The second edition of the *Handbook* (1956), edited by Janet Doe and Mary Louise Marshall [2], updated the one-volume first edition, retaining whenever possible the original chapter authors. The preface to this volume included an apology for publication delays and noted that some of the information in the volume was written three or more years prior to publication.

Fourteen years elapsed before the third edition, the first one published by MLA, appeared in 1970. Editors Gertrude L. Annan and Jacqueline W. Felter took an entirely different approach: "The chapters are written by a new cadre of authors and differ from those of the earlier edition in substance and emphasis" [3]. Despite the expansion of the scope and coverage, the one-volume format was retained. Four consultants from different types of health sciences libraries ensured that the content took into account library practice in these settings. Publication delays continued to be a problem and were

> of grave concern to the editors who regret that some chapters were written several years before the volume went to press. With so many involved in the preparation of the work, unforeseen emergencies arose which prevented its production in the period scheduled [4].

Louise Darling, David Bishop, and Lois Ann Colaianni edited the fourth edition, published between 1982 and 1988. This edition included a "shift in terminology from medical to health science libraries . . . in itself . . . indicative of the new complexity, the highly interdisciplinary nature of the fields served by these libraries" [5]. However, the title of the *Handbook* was not changed "because of the risk of obscuring the continuity of editions" [6]. A three-volume format was chosen to "accommodate material on new developments, lessen the delays inherent in a multiple-author work, and facilitate later revision" [7]. This new approach did not, however, prevent publication delays:

> Even with a smaller number of authors per volume, the considerable time difference in submission of chapters has meant that the problem of keeping material within the volume on the same level of currency, though reduced, has not been solved [8].

In addition, "the sequential publication has resulted in problems of uneven currency in the completed work" [9]. "A more satisfactory method for revising the *Handbook* in the future is now under study, as the rapid pace of change in the information field obviously requires a new approach" [10].

In 1989, the MLA Books Panel recommended that the *Handbook* be continued with the same general scope and content as the fourth edition but that the three volumes be further divided into a series of smaller monographs, each dealing with a single subject and each with its own volume editor. An editor in chief, assisted by an Advisory Committee, was appointed to coordinate the publication. The Advisory Committee determined that health sciences librarianship is changing so rapidly that the profession will be better served by publication of a series and that the series required a new title. In this way, individual volumes can be updated as needed, without having to wait for the completion of all volumes in an edition, and the individual volumes will have a greater identity as independent books.

CPHSL will appear in eight volumes. The editors or authors of each volume are noted here:

Volume 1: Reference and Information Services in Health Sciences Libraries, M. Sandra Wood, editor

Volume 2: Educational Services in Health Sciences Libraries, Francesca
　Allegri, editor
Volume 3: Information Access and Delivery in Health Sciences Libraries,
　Carolyn Lipscomb, editor
*Volume 4: Collection Development and Assessment in Health Sciences Li-
braries,* by Daniel T. Richards and Dottie Eakin
Volume 5: Acquisitions in Health Sciences Libraries, David Morse, editor
*Volume 6: Bibliographic Management of Information Resources in Health
Sciences Libraries,* Laurie L. Thompson, editor
*Volume 7: Health Sciences Environment and Librarianship in Health Sci-
ences Libraries,* Lucretia W. McClure, editor
Volume 8: Administration and Management in Health Sciences Libraries,
　Rick B. Forsman, editor

The editor in chief is extremely fortunate in being able to tap the expertise of a group of very talented and dedicated MLA members as advisers, editors, and chapter authors. The *CPHSL* Advisory Committee provided valuable advice on the organization and content of *CPHSL,* recommended a
publication plan and timetable, and assisted in the identification of editors
and chapter authors.

The editors have total responsibility for the preparation for publication of
their volume, including selection of authors, review of content and adherence to established style and format guidelines, and maintenance of the publication schedule. Authors were asked to include in their chapters, as applicable, the following considerations: ethics, standards, legal aspects, staffing
issues and implications, differing practices as they apply to different types of
libraries, research, evaluation, technology/automation, and budgeting and
financing.

An extensive expert review process involved both academic and hospital
librarians. Each volume includes a listing of the expert reviewers of that volume, in grateful acknowledgment of their efforts. The editor in chief and the
editors are indebted to two of MLA's managing editors of books, J. Michael
Homan and Beryl Glitz, for selecting reviewers and coordinating their work
and for making personal suggestions on organization, content, and format.

Volumes 1-5 of *CPHSL* were copublished by the Medical Library Association and Scarecrow Press. Special thanks are due to David B. Biesel, director
of Scarecrow's Association Publishing Program; Raymond S. Naegele, MLA's
director of financial and administrative services; and Kimberly S. Pierceall,
MLA's director of communications for their advice and assistance during the
preparation of these volumes. From 1998 to 1999, MLA had a copublishing
agreement with Forbes Custom Publishing. Forbes published volume 7. In
1999 contracts were signed with Scarecrow Press for volumes 6 and 8 of the

series. The indexing expertise of Beryl Glitz provides consistent and accurate access to the content of each volume.

Alison Bunting, Editor in Chief
Louise M. Darling Biomedical Library
University of California, Los Angeles

REFERENCES

1. Doe J, Ed. Handbook of medical library practice. Chicago: American Library Association, 1942:v.

2. Doe J, Marshall, ML, eds. Handbook of medical library practice. 2nd ed. Chicago: American Library Association, 1956.

3. Annan GL, Felter JW, eds. Handbook of medical library practice. 3rd ed. Chicago: Medical Library Association, 1970:v.

4. Ibid., vii.

5. Darling L, Bishop D, Colaianni LA, eds. Handbook of medical library practice. 4th ed. v. 1. Chicago: Medical Library Association, 1982:xi.

6. Ibid.

7. Ibid., xii.

8. Darling L, Bishop D, Colaianni LA, eds. Handbook of medical library practice. 4th ed. v. 3. Chicago: Medical Library Association, 1988: xiv.

9. Ibid.

10. Ibid., xv.

Expert Reviewers

David W. Boilard, Toledo, OH
Frances A. Brahmi, Indianapolis, IN
Karen Brewer, New York, NY
Gary D. Byrd, Buffalo, NY
Anna Beth Crabtree, Springfield, MO
Susan N. Craft, Casper, WY
Diana J. Cunningham, Valhalla, NY
Rosalind F. Dudden, Denver, CO
Nelson J. Gilman, Los Angeles, CA
Mary E. Helms, Omaha, NE
Alice K. Kawakami, Los Angeles, CA
Regina Kenny Marone, New Haven, CT
Michelynn McKnight, Norman, OK
Faith A. Meakin, Gainesville, FL
Peggy Mullay-Quijas, Kansas City, MO
T. Scott Plutchak, Birmingham, AL
Virginia G. Saha, Cleveland, OH
Valerie Su, Stanford, CA
Carolyn G. Weaver, Seattle, WA
Thomas L. Williams, Mobile, AL

Advisory Committee Members

Rachael K. Anderson
Director, Arizona Health Sciences Center Library
University of Arizona
Tucson, AZ

Alison Bunting
Associate University Librarian for Sciences
Louise M. Darling Biomedical Library
University of California, Los Angeles
Los Angeles, CA

Dottie Eakin
Director
(1989-2000)
Medical Sciences Library
Texas A&M University
College Station, TX

Rick B. Forsman
Director, Denison Memorial Library
University of Colorado Health Sciences Center
Denver, CO

Ruth Holst
Director of Library Services
Medical Library
Columbia Hospital
Milwaukee, WI

J. Michael Homan
Director of Libraries
Mayo Foundation
Rochester, MN

Mary Horres
Associate University Librarian for Sciences
(1982-1998)
Biomedical Library
University of California, San Diego
La Jolla, CA

M. Sandra Wood
Librarian, Reference and Database Services
George T. Harrell Library
Milton S. Hershey Medical Center
Pennsylvania State University
Hershey, PA

Authors

Joan S. Ash
Associate Professor
Biomedical Information & Communication Center
Oregon Health Sciences University
Portland, OR

Prudence W. Dalrymple
Dean and Associate Professor
Graduate School of Library and Information Science
Dominican University
River Forest, IL

Ellen G. Detlefsen
Associate Professor, School of Information Sciences
University of Pittsburgh
Pittsburgh, PA

Barbara A. Epstein
Associate Director, Health Sciences Library System
University of Pittsburgh
Pittsburgh, PA

Rick B. Forsman
Director, Denison Memorial Library
University of Colorado Health Sciences Center
Denver, CO

Carol Jenkins
Director, Health Sciences Library
University of North Carolina
Chapel Hill, NC

Patricia C. Mickelson
Director, Health Sciences Library System
University of Pittsburgh
Pittsburgh, PA

Lynn Kasner Morgan
Director, Gustave L. and Janet W. Levy Library
Mount Sinai School of Medicine
New York, NY

Audrey Powderly Newcomer
Director, Health Sciences Center Library
Saint Louis University
St. Louis, MO

Mary Joan (M.J.) Tooey
Deputy Director
Health Sciences and Human Services Library
University of Maryland
Baltimore, MD

Frieda O. Weise
Executive Director
Health Sciences and Human Services Library
University of Maryland
Baltimore, MD

Elizabeth H. Wood
Head of Research and Reference Services
Health Sciences Library
Oregon Health Sciences University
Portland, OR

Introduction

A dozen years have passed since the third volume of the *Handbook of Medical Library Practice* provided an overview of administrative topics [1]. Management fads have come and gone during that period, but the basic elements of operating a library remain fairly constant. The astute administrator must apply basic management concepts in a specialized setting, allocating resources for the efficient operation of the library and the delivery of high-quality information services. As described by chapter authors in the current volume, the library director's work has broadened to include new tasks in some institutions. At the same time, the complexity of each set of tasks has increased due to new technology and legal requirements and expectations of accountability that have grown over time.

This volume does not purport to be a comprehensive, stand-alone treatise on health sciences library administration. The reader will also need to refer to both the general literature of management and that of library management. Each chapter provides a synopsis of a particular aspect of health sciences library management; taken together, they give a balanced overview of the key tasks faced by the manager. The chapters are intended for practical application by a working library practitioner rather than being theoretical discussions.

Today health sciences libraries sit midstream in a rapid and unpredictable period of change as technology transforms services, staffing, and physical facilities. This is one of the most dynamic and exciting times to practice in the field! Accordingly, a constant theme throughout this volume is the necessity for the library director to actively reshape the role, priorities, and supporting operations of the library. Blessed with an array of powerful new technological tools, health sciences librarians will once again lead the profession in introducing cutting-edge products and services.

The editor and authors of this volume hope that readers will find the content a useful touchstone and practical primer as they reconsider and transfigure their libraries. In *A Midsummer Night's Dream,* Shakespeare said that change and confusion occur, "[s]wift as a shadow, short as a dream/[b]rief as the lightening in the collied night" [2]. Libraries have become lightning rods for technological and organizational change, with the director seeking a path through an environment replete with confusion, uncertainty, and urgency. This introduction is intentionally brief so the reader, ever more pressed for time, may proceed apace to the pragmatic knowledge distilled in these chapters.

Rick B. Forsman
Denver, Colorado

REFERENCES

1. Darling L, Bishop D, Colaianni LA, eds. Handbook of medical library practice. 4th ed. v. 3. Chicago: Medical Library Association, 1988.
2. Familiar quotations by John Bartlett. 13th ed. Boston, Little, Brown: 1955:141a.

Management Challenges in an Era of Change: An Overview

Barbara A. Epstein, Patricia C. Mickelson, and Ellen G. Detlefsen

Change is a constant factor in human existence, but the pace of change is accelerating. Rapid advances in technological development create both unprecedented opportunities and enormous dilemmas for library managers in health care settings, whether they work in small hospital libraries or large academic medical centers. The impact of information technologies, including the Internet, expert systems for both diagnosis and therapy, new methods and systems for institution-wide communications, and the proliferation of computer-based tools for care, are dramatically changing the physical environment and the culture of medical institutions. Similarly, faster computers, advanced networking technology, and the growing availability of full-text digital information transform the library's goal of providing full information directly to the patient's bedside or the researcher's workstation from a dream to an achievable objective.

The introduction of new services quickly leads to rising user expectations for additional services, creating extraordinary pressure on budgets and staffs that may not grow as quickly as user demands. Library managers face competition for limited institutional resources, yet at the same time they struggle with shrinking buying power and a proliferation of resources for sale in a variety of print and digital formats. The perception that time is literally moving faster creates an atmosphere in which managers feel pressured to act quickly, with little time for lengthy deliberation or long-term planning. How did this sense of urgency come about, and how should health sciences library administrators respond?

HEALTH CARE IN THE NEW MILLENNIUM

Even a casual review of recent headlines and news reports reveals that health care is undergoing radical and rapid change with the goal of controlling costs and modifying delivery structures [1]. Simply stated, it seems likely that the nation's and the world's economies will no longer support the high costs of providing health care within the traditional fee-for-service reimbursement structure. Various plans for reforming health care have been proposed, but no consensus has yet developed about what constitutes the best system.

A number of trends, however, have emerged that will guide the discussion of health care planning in coming years, and they already have had a dramatic effect on health sciences libraries and those who administer them. Not only must library managers be aware of these trends, they must be able to act on them as they impact the larger institutions in which the unit under management finds itself. The successful manager will see these changes as opportunities for increased institution-wide integration and not as insurmountable or discouraging impediments. Strong management skills will enable library administrators to succeed in this volatile environment.

This shift to a managed care philosophy relies on capitated systems of reimbursement replacing fee-based systems. Health care providers are increasingly compensated based on the number of insured lives in their care rather than the number of procedures they perform. Hospitals are receiving reduced third-party reimbursements for patient care and thus are pursuing aggressive cost containment. In many areas, health care facilities compete fiercely for patients, particularly those who are well insured. Institutional units that cannot cover their own costs or that are seen as a financial drain on the parent institution may be eliminated or drastically curtailed. In this milieu, libraries in particular may face the real risk of being perceived as luxurious anachronisms replaceable by hardware and software run by end users, such as clinicians and researchers working with integrated information systems at their desks and in their clinical examination rooms.

To compete for managed care contracts, achieve economies of scale, and enhance their bargaining power with insurance companies, hospitals join forces with one another and with other facilities to create health care conglomerates offering "one-stop shopping" for consumers. Shortell, Gillies, and Devers [2] argue persuasively that hospitals will no longer function as the core delivery mechanism of American health care, as the inpatient-oriented illness model of health care is replaced with one focused on disease prevention and health promotion. They assert that "the likely success of this effort will depend on the hospital's ability to reinvent and in some respects, 'lose' itself within a network of organized, community-oriented health and social service delivery systems focused on broad aspects of health care and chronic disease management" [3].

Mergers of widely divergent health care facilities create complex systems that include primary, secondary, and tertiary health care facilities. The organizational structures of these systems can change at such a rapid rate that the power structures and decision-making mechanisms may be unclear, even to its own employees. Hospitals that merge into such systems often face major restructuring of their services. Libraries appear particularly vulnerable to these forces because of the possible duplication of services that occurs when institutional mergers and takeovers combine facilities with multiple existing libraries. Emerging health care systems may include several similar-sized hospital libraries, or—if an academic medical center or medical school is involved—a large academic health sciences library and one or more hospital libraries. This creates the necessity for new cooperative relationships and re-examination of service philosophies, collection development, and possibly reporting structures. Library managers must be attentive to both institutional and systemwide priorities and open to opportunities that arise in the shifting organizational structure.

Decreased utilization of hospital facilities is leading to shorter inpatient stays, earlier discharge into the community, and the concomitant increased use of home health care and skilled nursing facilities. With a decrease in inpatient censuses, the traditional library functions of supporting the hospital-based delivery of clinical care must shift to providing information to support the outpatient services that may be delivered in scattered facilities miles from the parent institution and the traditional library. These services may also extend to the inclusion of patient education and consumer information services that support expanded outpatient care.

Increased emphasis on preventive care, to keep people healthy and out of the hospital, leads naturally to an increased emphasis on consumer education, with patients taking more responsibility for remaining healthy. Consumers are bombarded with drug advertisements and other health information in magazines and newspapers, on television, and via the Internet. Research results from mainstream and respected medical journals are reported on the evening news, not always in accurate detail. But busy clinicians often have less time to spend with patients to interpret or explain such information; hence, the demand for accurate and definitive consumer information grows, along with the need for standards to identify such information.

Librarians have an opportunity to become full team members in a new consumer health-oriented environment, but they must move aggressively lest these services be assigned or delegated to other providers in the institution. A number of other health professionals—notably pharmacists, nurses, social workers, and health educators—are actively pursuing new roles in the provision of consumer- (or "family-" or "patient-") focused information. The librarian's professional commitment to open access to a wide range of information and ideas may be at odds with clinicians unused to well-informed and questioning patients. Cautious administrators may be wary of patient misunderstandings and possible litigation. The notion of a team approach to clinical care mandates that librarians find ways to demonstrate the value of their presence in clinical teams, especially those devoted to outpatient services where libraries have had little prior impact and involvement.

Cost containment encourages a shift from specialist to generalist physicians, and to the increased use of primary care providers other than physicians, such as nurse practitioners and physician assistants. In managed care environments, family practitioners, pediatricians, gynecologists, and other primary care physicians (PCPs) function as gatekeepers. Patients must be referred to specialists by their PCP, or they face high out-of-pocket fees if they seek care without the gatekeeper's permission. There is likewise an increasing use of nurse practitioners and physician assistants to provide primary and preventive health care.

The information needs and behaviors of PCPs and care providers other than physicians are not well documented, but research suggests that their practices will require access to a variety of integrated information resources, including clinical information repositories, "knowledge-based" information available through the library, and other resources. Most information behavior research has focused on academic physicians and physicians in training. These groups exhibit a strong need for both knowledge-based and patient-specific information, but they apparently choose to acquire the knowledge most often from gatekeeper colleagues, personal files, old textbooks, and only sometimes from libraries [4-7]. There is less systematic research on the information behaviors of other groups of health professionals and very little research that looks at these behaviors in a managed care environment [8].

Reduced support for training of health professionals, as mandated in the Balanced Budget Act of 1997 [9], results in budgetary pressure for academic medical centers to place a greater emphasis on direct patient care. At the same time, the formation of health care systems, including academic health centers and community facilities, combined with the movement to train more primary care providers, result in students circulating throughout the system [10]. Libraries and library managers will have to find effective ways of extending library resources to students and health care professionals in off-site, rotating, and often remote locations. Simply put, the challenge for libraries is to provide more information to more diverse users in more places.

At the national level, practice guidelines, clinical pathways, and similar evidence-based tools are increasingly being implemented to combine quality and consistency in cost-effective treatment methodologies across different health facilities. Within institutions and systems, clinical pathways determine the optimal levels of care delivered by institutional personnel. Similarly, education in medicine and other health professions is shifting away from memorization and rote learning to emphasize problem-based learning (PBL), wherein students are challenged to work in groups to find answers to real-life problems. Sophisticated clinicians who have adopted evidence-based practice (EBP) are especially dependent on information services at their desktops and fingertips. They search for fact-based evidence reported in clinical trials in order to make clinical decisions. As key participants in information delivery, librarians are frequently involved in EBP projects [11-12]. The information-intensive nature of PBL and the evidence-based medical environment challenge medical libraries to develop better instructional methods to teach users how to retrieve and apply knowledge-based information. Those who manage collections of information must be able to position resources and personnel in ways which optimize its use.

The emerging field of telehealth serves as one example of how a new medical specialty creates major demands from several sectors. Telehealth clinicians and tertiary specialists want immediate access at any time, day or night, to full-text tools and complex imaging and telecommunications programs. At the University of Iowa, the National Laboratory for the Study of Rural Telemedicine is a leader in using technology to provide health care and health information to an isolated rural environment with a dispersed population, overburdened hospital systems and public health services, and professionally isolated health care providers [13]. These needs expand to a global arena as domestic U.S. health care systems link up with international partners [14]. Telehealth has even been hailed as a cost-effective method— cheaper than international travel, fax, or telephone—for providing clinical and consultative services to Europe, Asia, and the emerging Third World [15]. Libraries can be the venue in which clinicians learn to master telehealth technology [16].

IMPACT OF TECHNOLOGY

The impact of technology on virtually every library process is described in detail in Chapter 5, The Technological Transformation of Health Sciences Libraries. The curatorial and archival role of the traditional library manager is giving way to new units and new roles as the manager for information in digital as well as textual formats. In many hospitals and academic centers, library managers find themselves competing for influence or resources with larger information systems (IS) departments responsible for clinical and financial information systems within the health center. Review or approval from the IS department may be necessary to purchase new hardware and software, and the library often relies on IS infrastructure and support services. This IS oversight and control can either foster collaboration or create interunit conflict. In some settings the library has great latitude to introduce emerging technologies, producing the same potential for cooperation or confrontation with the IS department.

Since standards [17] of the Joint Commission on Accreditation of Healthcare Organizations (JCAHO) treat "access to knowledge-based information" (i.e., books, journals, and databases traditionally provided by libraries) as simply another facet of information provision within the hospital, library managers often serve on information management committees. These present crucial opportunities for the library manager to communicate library capabilities and needs, to form political alliances, and to position the library advantageously [18-19].

In 1982 Matheson and Cooper first envisioned Integrated Advanced Information Management Systems [20]. In today's larger health care organizations, such IAIMS projects present opportunities for libraries to plan and partner with managers of hospital clinical information systems, educational specialists, offices of research, and departments of informatics. Librarians may find themselves working closely with other IAIMS professionals with the goal of integrating the library's "knowledge-based" information with patient care information and decision support systems accessible on a single workstation.

Due to the focus on information management in health centers, reorganization of departments and changes in reporting structures are occurring. Restructuring may result in an expanded role for the library and its staff [21]. The library may manage academic computing functions or have primary responsibility for networking activities on a health sciences campus [22]. In either a clinical or academic setting, the health sciences library may become part of a large information management unit and report to a chief information officer [23]. In some instances, the librarian may herself become the chief information officer [24]. In any event, sensitivity to the political environment and the strategic goals of the institution are essential for successfully negotiating the rapidly changing environment.

The fast pace of technological innovation can result in the need for libraries to run simultaneous systems of traditional services and new technologies during a lengthy transition period, and it requires library managers to wrestle with library staffing issues as well as with user training issues. The lead time available to research, evaluate, install, and update new systems is shrinking. Staff feel pressure to learn new systems more quickly, not only for their own use but also to train end users and offer troubleshooting assistance. In very concrete terms, consider that MEDLINE training for librarians took six months in the late 1960s, yet the training time for end users in many institutions shrank to less than one hour by the late 1990s. Many users consider themselves able to conduct basic searches of the PubMed database (available on the Internet from the National Library of Medicine) with no formal training at all. Current library staff members require frequent training and skills updating to cope with continual computer enhancements, and new hires must already possess the skills to use information technologies efficiently and effectively.

THE CHALLENGE OF CHANGE

The changes outlined in the prior sections create new service demands, many of which resulted from the advent of new information products. High-speed telecommunications, vastly more efficient computing, and user feelings of entitlement to universal access have changed the nature of client behavior. Clients expect to be able to do more because they have been trained in faster work methods that take advantage of office and desktop computing. Their expectations make it mandatory for library managers to mount or coordinate bigger, better, and faster information environments from the library. Needs assessment, planning and implementation of new services and systems must occur proactively, as users will not be satisfied with the status quo for very long. At the same time, users with more traditional viewpoints or those who are unfamiliar with or who do not have access to up-to-date hardware in their immediate work area may resist new technology.

It has become increasingly difficult to remain abreast of new technology and to determine whether the new products actually add value or only automate functions of questionable worth. Library staff need to be conversant with both technical and administrative issues to evaluate emerging technology. Library managers must set aside time and money—both precious commodities—for personal and staff education and training in the selection and implementation of new technologies.

The complexity of licensing electronic resources can be one of the most daunting administrative tasks today. Library managers sometimes find themselves serving as educators both of the publisher/vendor who is unfamiliar with their specific institutional environment and institutional purchasing agents and legal counsel who may be unfamiliar with the complexities of leased digital information resources. Given the fast pace of development, the latest information about licensing issues is often found on the Internet [25-26]. Access management and authentication issues in the rapidly evolving technological and institutional environment pose complex issues [27]. Lack of clear industry standards, publisher inexperience with user behavior in the digital environment, uncertainty about archiving policies, the difficulty of calculating the need for simultaneous user licenses, and a myriad of other issues make this uncharted territory both for library managers and vendor/publishers. The library manager must develop a basic knowledge of contract law and business practices as related to this new industry and form a working relationship with the institution's legal counsel.

Change also heightens expectations of the institution's administration. Some administrators want their libraries to deliver complete information from the Internet, without fully understanding the complexities of transforming a print environment to a digital one. These bosses ask plaintively or aggressively, "Why should we pay when we can get all this for free on the Web?" Or they want to know, "Why do we still buy journals if they're all online?" Currently, hospitals are not mandated by JCAHO or other regulatory agencies to maintain library collections and staffs as long as they can demonstrate that access to knowledge-based information is provided via online systems or contracts with other health care facilities. Consequently, librarians may be forced to justify their very existence every year at budget time. Successful library managers will be able to educate their institutional administrators about reasonable expectations while firing their imaginations about services that could be provided by the library if given adequate resources.

Changing economic conditions create numerous perplexing fiscal challenges. The inflation rate for printed materials, especially scientific and medical journals, continues to be well above the general cost-of-living rate [28-31]. At the same time, the rapid pace of technological development demands ever more powerful software, hardware, and systems networks that require new infusions of capital into already weakened library budgets. While many libraries are progressing rapidly toward the achievement of the concept of a "digital library," few have been able to reduce costs or cancel print subscriptions as a result of automating functions or offering full-text electronic materials. Difficult questions about pricing policies, copyright, archiving, and licensing must be resolved between libraries and the publishing industry before significant savings can occur. Library managers must assertively negotiate with administrators to acquire the resources necessary to carry out their mission. (See also Chapter 2, Fiscal Management in Health Sciences Libraries, in this volume.)

Educators of health professionals are also clamoring for information services, especially user training and outreach programs. Health sciences librarians are serving more frequently as trainers and facilitators in the problem-based learning curricula that are increasingly popular in medical schools. One of the hallmarks of PBL is an emphasis on information management [32-33]. Students in a PBL curriculum—even if in only a partial PBL environment—learn from day one that access to, and the appropriate use of, information is essential to careful and cost-effective medical practice [34]. Librarians are also playing increasingly larger roles in the provision of distance learning experiences for nursing education and in-service continuing education for clinicians. Educators in the health professions are the natural partners for librarians in this effort to train the next generation of health professionals. As a result, library managers in academic settings are faced with competing demands for their reference and education staff members' time.

Hospital librarians experience similar pressures. Of particular note are the changing expectations for small libraries garnered from health professionals who obtained their degrees and training at large system-based health care institutions with excellent access to electronic technology. When these professionals enter practice settings, they bring with them the experiences of their education, and they expect the small hospital library and its manager to provide the same levels of service, sophisticated technology, and speedy access that they enjoyed in their training years.

The medical research community—whether in the basic sciences or in clinical research—needs more information and more information services support to conduct its work. Advances in the fields of genetics, molecular biology and biotechnology hold the potential to revolutionize the treatment, diagnosis, and prevention of disease. Researchers in these fields may use large "libraries" of genome information or extensive files of longitudinal patient data. They require both access to and training in the use of these non-bibliographic databases, and they may expect the library to be their source for both. Similarly, there is an urgent need to educate physicians about genetics advances, so these can be integrated into clinical medicine [35]. Thus, research consultation services may be added to the portfolio of the reference staff in medical libraries, resulting in the need to hire or develop librarians with very specialized knowledge and skills. The inevitable tension between the high costs of access to these research files versus the need for comprehensiveness in order to satisfy a broad range of user needs results in a management challenge.

ADMINISTRATIVE RESPONSE: BLENDING TRADITION WITH INNOVATION

Based on the dynamics of the trends and challenges outlined here, it is clear that the next five to ten years will mandate significant and unforeseeable changes in the health care environment and in the libraries that will survive to serve these institutions. Those who administer these libraries will have to make major adjustments in their own vision and expectations. Library managers must critically and periodically reevaluate their administrative structures, service delivery mechanisms, collection development, computer systems, budget allocation, staffing patterns, and physical space to adapt to their new institutional environment. How many "directors of library services" can a multihospital health system accommodate? Can "behind-the-scenes" functions such as technical services and interlibrary loan be centralized? Can reference staff in one location serve multiple sites? Is the electronic mail system adequate for communication with clinicians at remote sites? Does every hospital need to store bound volumes of medical journals, or can the subscription be available online throughout the system? Does every hospital need a "library space," or will online systems with email assistance suffice? Should the cost of online systems be allocated to individual units or calculated into overhead costs? Should the print collection be eliminated altogether but the librarian retained? The answers to these and similar questions vary with each institution but require clear-headed and objective consideration and a willingness to let go of familiar methods of operation to venture into new territory.

To arrive at credible and persuasive solutions to the challenges described here, the library administrator must use both proven and emerging management techniques. The body of management literature has proliferated as theorists and academicians attempt to forecast and describe social changes and advocate proactive and adaptive responses. Much of this writing is in the field traditionally labeled "business" or "business administration," and popular authors and terminology can easily be identified. Braude's 1989 work stands as a comprehensive summary of the basic principles of management as applied to health sciences libraries [36]. We do not intend to summarize the literature of management; rather, we encourage the reader to review materials listed in the references to this chapter as well as literature on general management, library management, and health sciences management. It is incumbent on the library manager, however, to consider judiciously how various management theories and ideas can be best applied in a real-life setting. While a plethora of "experts" offer advice and the "solution du jour," there is no substitute for common sense and firsthand knowledge of the environment and the situation.

PREPARING STAFF FOR NEW ROLES

In larger libraries, designing an efficient and effective organizational structure challenges any director. Traditional hierarchical arrangements have given way to flatter organizational structures with fewer levels between the top and the bottom. Work teams, task forces, and other flexible groups bring together workers from traditionally separate areas, such as technical services, reference, and systems, to accomplish the complex tasks necessary in this fast-paced environment. Although management guru Tom Peters has stated, "If you aren't reorganizing, pretty substantially, once every six to twelve months, you're probably out of step with the times" [37], the prudent manager should try to retain enough stability in the organization to anchor the staff through turbulent times. Gaius Petronius's description of a period of rapid change in the Roman Empire remains valid:

> We trained hard to meet our challenges, but it seemed as if every time we were beginning to form into teams we would be re-organized. I was to learn later in

life that we tend to meet any new situation by reorganizing; and a wonderful method it can be for creating the illusion of progress while producing confusion, ineffectiveness and demoralization [38].

Another of the requirements of the library manager's changing role is the ability to work with and lead people who know more about technology than the manager does. Professional staff in the library may include computer systems analysts and others with advanced degrees in computer or information sciences. The job of managing such experts is a relatively new role for librarians, who may be more comfortable with the management of individuals who are trained as they were and who know well the traditional world of library practice. Of particular note is the issue of managing equitable salary distribution when the marketplace may compensate the technological expert with an associate or bachelor's degree at a higher level than the librarian with a master's degree. A companion problem is in the integration of technological experts in the community of library practice when these individuals may have no understanding of, or appreciation for, the traditions, customary service orientation, and other values of the library world.

Of particular interest is the need for all library staff members, not just the degreed librarians, to learn to be managers. Public services librarians must manage departments that involve both traditional reference desk services and heavy teaching responsibilities. Technical services librarians must manage outsourcing contracts, paraprofessional staff, and commercial relationships with vendors, producers, and publishers. Personnel in media centers and computer facilities must manage changing technologies, depreciation and replacement of systems, and high turnover of technical staff. These individuals will need assistance and managerial support to make the obligatory transition from a traditional library role into that of a self-directed "knowledge manager" in an integrated information management environment [39]. If this individual is herself the library manager, she must look both within herself and also persuade her immediate supervisor to provide the freedom and financial support to move ahead.

Notable, perhaps, as a first area of concern for new leadership, is the area of financial control. The need for expertise in fiscal management has become critical. Managers are required to make stable or shrinking funding go farther. Necessary fiscal decisions within one's own library and institution, as well as in interdepartmental collaborations and resource-sharing relationships, force managers to learn new ways of handling fiscal resources. Skill with spreadsheets, budget projection software, and decision making under uncertainty are now a necessary part of the manager's abilities.

Similarly, new skills in salesmanship, marketing, and promotion are required to position the library as a team player in the new health care environment. Communication, marketing, public relations, and training occupy an increasingly important and time-consuming role in the library manager's work life (see also Chapter 4, Marketing Library Services, in this volume). The ability to explain and promote information services effectively to a clientele with varying levels of acceptance and information literacy is vital. This means not only the ability to sell traditional library services to those who do not currently use them but also to showcase new areas of information expertise such as Internet-based services. Librarians must be able to catch the attention of users who are pressed for time and resources and demonstrate quickly and convincingly how the library's automated systems can make their job easier. Newsletters, home pages, bulletin boards, displays, formal classes, informal consultations—all become necessary tools in communicating the library's purpose and services. Writing, speaking, and promotional skills have never been as important. Outreach services must be managed in a manner that will attract new users, while the organization continues to retain existing users.

Another area of managerial concern is time allocation. Librarians and library managers seek new leadership roles to enhance their professional credibility and visibility, but these roles also require more work. Training and professional development experiences will be necessary to become expert in crucial new management areas. As managers juggle their traditional responsibilities with the need to move into new roles, they must carefully balance the advantages of taking on enhanced duties within the larger institution against the necessity of maintaining everyday library operations. Of course, some formerly time-consuming jobs may be delegated or phased out. In the long run, however, it may be ultimately self-defeating, though tempting, to accept a myriad of new assignments without being assured of extra resources to accomplish core responsibilities or identifying outdated tasks that can be eliminated. Individuals drawn to service organizations often find it easy to take on added tasks but have difficulty in identifying responsibilities they can relinquish.

RESPONDING THROUGH PROFESSIONAL DEVELOPMENT AND EDUCATION

Library staff and managers have to learn faster, be self-directed, and take personal and professional responsibility for their own life-long learning. Such an approach is outlined in the Medical Library Association's *Platform for Change* document, which stresses the responsibility of the individual member to identify areas for professional development [40]. Such personal efforts are rewarded through membership at various levels in the Association's Academy of Health Information Professionals. The traditional concept of an annual, day-long continuing education course taken while attending a national or regional conference is changing rapidly, as individuals and libraries find that it is temporally and fiscally impossible to support such a model. The continuing education programs of the Medical Library Association and other organizations have expanded greatly. They now incorporate World Wide Web–based tutorials, learning contracts, continuing education credit for programs offered outside of meetings, internships, apprenticeships, sabbaticals for the pursuit of formal degrees, in-house inservice seminars, teleconferences, and industry-based corporate educational packages, as well as traditional classroom-based learning in formal graduate library and information science programs.

The set of new skills required to function and manage in this environment is difficult to project over the long run. Several recent research efforts have attempted to codify critical skills and competencies that library managers should seek to enhance in both their own and their staff members' professional development. In May 1989, the Task Force on Knowledge and Skills of the Medical Library Association identified seven broad areas in which health information professionals should possess varying levels of knowledge and skills [41]. In 1996, the Special Library Association issued a report defining competencies viewed as essential for members to master [42]. In 1997, research projects at Vanderbilt University [43] and the University of Pittsburgh [44] surveyed health sciences librarians and library users to identify skills currently necessary and those perceived to be necessary in the future. These are listed in Appendix A of this volume. These lists of prescribed skills call for a complex blend of overlapping personal and professional attributes whose pursuit can strain the professional development resources of even the most dedicated library manager.

A further question arises: Even if librarians master these new skills, will they then be ready to step into the leadership vacuum and provide guidance in areas hitherto not their forte or even their "turf"? The myriad issues that surround the licensing of intellectual property and access to distributed electronic resources described earlier already press library managers to develop new skills in the legal and negotiating arenas, yet most librarians have no formal legal education.

A related area is the need to recruit talented newcomers into the field. The National Library of Medicine's onetime round of planning grants for the education and training of health sciences librarians resulted in several new models for the delivery of professional education, continuing education, and internships [45-51]. A problem of recruiting individuals with a science or health science background has also been identified [52]. Some model programs for recruitment at the high school and undergraduate levels have been attempted, but little success has yet been achieved. Consequently, recruitment of the "best and brightest" remains a problematic issue for the profession.

BECOMING A RISK TAKER

A final challenge is that of becoming risk taker, particularly as the manager works to reengineer structures outside of and also within the library. Just as clinicians learn to make life-and-death decisions without complete information—the problem that physicians have labeled "reasoning under uncertainty"—so librarians must work in a stressful world of decision making where risk is both personal and institutional. As Walter Wriston, former chairman of Citibank, once noted, "Good judgment is the result of experience, and experience is the result of bad judgment" [53].

> What the manager needs today is not management theory or the pedagogy of business school professors. . . . Today's manager needs the old verities: vision, judgment, reflexes, conviction. And the modern ones: good data and the fastest tools [54].

Sweeping changes in the health care environment coupled with dramatic technological advances in recent years have resulted in unique opportunities and challenges for the library administrator. Satisfying new service demands, incorporating new technology, maintaining a sound budget in an era of shrinking resources, reinventing the role of the librarian, recruiting and retaining staff with specialized skills, reengineering the library organization, and generally thriving in the turbulent new health care environment all require that the library manager have a rich resource of management skills to draw upon. Pursuing a graduate degree in business, health or public administration, or even law is not always a feasible route by which to acquire advanced management training, though it is the traditional educational pathway to gaining management credentials. Those who would acquire these skills on their own must seek a balanced array of experiences, short courses and continuing education activities, and appropriate mentoring in management. Disciplined reading and on-the-job exposure to managerial life are also useful.

Few clear-cut rules exist for attaining success as a manager during times of rapid and pervasive change. Instead, a mix of knowledge and skills is essential. An understanding of management principles and theories, coupled with knowledge of the institutional environment, a strong working relationship with other units in the institution, effective personal communication skills, well-developed political skills, good judgment, and the ability to flourish in a dynamic environment constitute a promising formula for a fruitful and rewarding management career.

REFERENCES

1. Freudenheim M. Medical insurers revise cost-control efforts. New York Times, Late Edition (East Coast) 1999 Dec 3: A1.

2. Shortell SM, Gillies RR, Devers KJ. Reinventing the American hospital. Milbank Q1995;73(2):131-60.

3. Ibid., 132.

4. Forsythe DE, et al. Expanding the concept of medical information: an observational study of physicians' information needs. Comput Biomed Res 1992;25(2):181-200.

5. Osheroff JA, et al. Physicians' information needs: analysis of questions posed during clinical teaching. Ann Intern Med 1991 Apr 1;114(7):576-81.

6. U.S. Agency for Health Care Policy and Research. Annotated bibliography: information dissemination to health care practitioners and policymakers. Rockville, MD: AHCPR, 1992. (AHCPR publication no. 92-0030)

7. Verhoeven AAH, Boerma EJ, Meyboom-de Jong B. Use of information sources by family physicians: a literature survey. Bull Med Lib Assoc 1995 Jan;83(1):85-90.

8. Detlefsen EG. The information behaviors of life and health scientists and health care providers: characteristics of the research literature. Bull Med Lib Assoc 1998 Jul;86(3):385-90.

9. Inglehart JK. Medicare and graduate medical education. N Engl J Med 1998 Feb 5;338(6):402-7.

10. Colwell JM, et al. Modifying the culture of medical education: the first three years of the RWJ Generalist Physician Initiative. Acad Med 1997 Sept;72(9):745-53.

11. McKibbon KA. Evidence-based practice. Bull Med Libr Assoc 1996 Jul;86(3):396-401.

12. McKibbon KA. Using "best evidence" in clinical practice. ACP J Club 1998;128(2):A15.

13. D'Alessandro MP, ed. Symposium: the University of Iowa digital library project. Bull Med Libr Assoc 1998 Oct;86(4):552-602.

14. Perednia DA, et al. Telemedicine technology and clinical applications. JAMA. 1995 Feb 8;273(6):483-8.

15. Wright D, et al. Telemedicine and developing countries. J Telemed Telecare 1996;2(2):63-70.

16. Zundel KM. Telemedicine: history, applications, and impact on librarianship. Bull Med Libr Assoc 1996 Jan;84(1):71-9.

17. Joint Commission on Accreditation of Healthcare Organizations. Comprehensive accreditation manual for hospitals. Oakbrook Terrace, IL: JCAHO, 1998.

18. Dalrymple PW, Scherrer CS. Tools for improvement: a systematic analysis and guide to accreditation by the JCAHO. Bull Med Libr Assoc 1998 Jan;86(1):10-6.

19. Glitz B, et al. Hospital library service and the changes in national standards. Bull Med Libr Assoc 1998 Jan;86(1):77-87.

20. Matheson NW, Cooper JA. Academic information in the academic health sciences center: roles for the library in information management. J Med Educ 1982 Oct;57(10, pt. 2):1-93.

21. Anderson RK, Fuller SS. Librarians as members of integrated institutional information programs: management and organizational issues. Libr Trends 1992;41(2):198-213.

22. Stead WW. Positioning the library at the epicenter of the networked biomedical enterprise. Bull Med Libr Assoc 1998 Jan;86(1):26-30.

23. Braude RM. Impact of information technology on the role of health sciences librarians. Bull Med Libr Assoc 1993 Oct;81(4):408-13.

24. Greer MC. The medical librarian as chief information officer. Bull Med Libr Assoc 1998 Jan;86(1):88-94.

25. Liblicense. Available from Internet: http://www.library.yale/~license.

26. Office of Scholarly Information, Association of Research Libraries, Washington, DC. Available from Internet: http://arl.cni.org/scomm/licensing.

27. Lynch C. Access management for networked information resources. Cause/Effect 1998;21(4) [online serial]. Available from Internet: http://www.educase.edu/ir/library/html/cem9842.html.

28. Brandon AN, Hill DR. Selected list of books and journals for the small medical library. Bull Med Libr Assoc 1997 Apr;85(2):111-35.

29. Hafner AW, et al. Journal pricing issues: an economic perspective. Bull Med Libr Assoc 1990 Jul;78(3):217-23.

30. Kronenfeld MR. Update on inflation of journal prices in the Brandon-Hill list of journals. Bull Med Libr Assoc 1996 Apr;84(2):260-3.

31. Index Medicus price study 1994-1998. Birmingham, AL: EBSCO Subscription Services, 1998.

32. Kanter SL. Fundamental concepts of problem-based learning for the new facilitator. Bull Med Libr Assoc 1998 Jul;86(3): 391-5.

33. Marshall JG, et al. A study of library use in problem-based and traditional medical curricula. Bull Med Libr Assoc 1993 Jul;81(3):299-305.

34. Schilling K, et al. Integration of information-seeking skills and activities into a problem-based curriculum. Bull Med Libr Assoc 1995 Apr;83(2):176-83.

35. Collins FS, Boch MK. Avoiding casualties in the genetic revolution: the urgent need to educate physicians about genetics. Acad Med 1999 Jan;74(1):48-9.

36. Braude RM. Administration: general principles applied to health science libraries. In: Darling L, Colaianni LA, Bishop D, eds. Handbook of medical library practice. 4th ed., v. 3. Chicago: Medical Library Association, 1988:221-85.

37. Peters T. Thriving on chaos: handbook for a management revolution. New York: Knopf, 1988:467.

38. Micklethwaite J, Wooldridge A. The witch doctors: making sense of the management gurus. New York: Times Books, 1996:326.

39. Matheson NW. The idea of the library in the twenty-first century. Bull Med Libr Assoc 1995 Jan;83(1):1-7.

40. Medical Library Association. Platform for change: the educational policy statement of the Medical Library Association. Chicago: Medical Library Association, 1992.

41. Ibid.

42. Special Libraries Association. Special Committee on Competencies for Special Librarians. Competencies for special librarians of the 21st Century. Washington, DC: Special Libraries Association, 1996.

43. Giuse NB, et al. Preparing librarians to meet the challenges of today's health care environment. J Am Med Inform Assoc 1997 Feb;4(1):57-67.

44. Detlefsen EG. Positioning yourself for the 21st century: career planning in a rapidly changing profession. Presentation for Philadelphia Regional Chapter, Medical Library Association, March 21, 1997.

45. Brandt KA, Sapp JR, Campbell JM. Current topics in health sciences librarianship: a pilot program for network-based lifelong learning. Bull Med Libr Assoc 1996 Oct;84(4):515-23.

46. Detlefsen EG, et al. Transforming the present—discovering the future: the University of Pittsburgh's NLM grant on education and training of health sciences librarians. Bull Med Libr Assoc 1996 Oct;84(4):524-33.

47. Giuse NB, et al. Integrating health sciences librarians into biomedicine. Bull Med Libr Assoc 1996 Oct;84(4):534-40.

48. Moran BB, et al. Preparing tomorrow's health sciences librarians: feasibility and marketing studies. Bull Med Libr Assoc 1996 Oct;84(4):541-8.

49. Roper FW, Barron DD, Funk CJ. Collaboration in a continuum of learning: developing the next generation of leadership. Bull Med Libr Assoc 1996 Oct;84(4):549-52.

50. Sievert MC, et al. The Missouri planning grant for the education and training of health sciences librarians. Bull Med Libr Assoc 1996 Oct;84(4):553-9.

51. Smith LC. Interdisciplinary multiinstitutional alliances in support of educational programs for health sciences librarians. Bull Med Libr Assoc 1996 Oct;84(4):560-8.

52. National Library of Medicine. Report of the Planning Panel on the Education and Training of Health Sciences Librarians. Bethesda, MD: National Library of Medicine, 1995.

53. Micklethwaite, op cit., 122.

54. Karlgaard R. Management theory in trouble. Forbes ASAP 1996;158(12):9.

2

Fiscal Management in Health Sciences Libraries

Lynn Kasner Morgan

The financial position of the parent institution affects all aspects of the health sciences library's ability to provide the organization with information services and resources. In the context of a U.S. health care system under scrutiny by government, industry, and consumers, library administrators face tremendous challenges in finding adequate financial means to support the traditional institutional missions of patient care, education, and research. Health care institutions, and hospitals in particular, are rightsizing, downsizing, privatizing, joining networks, being purchased, undergoing revised reimbursement methods, and being viewed as cost centers rather than profit centers in a changeable managed care environment [1]. Faced with massive and global changes in the health care system and the way it is financed, library administrators practicing in this milieu must be resourceful and creative in seeking adequate funds to meet the many demands placed on the library.

The health sciences librarian needs to know how to develop, present, and lobby for adequate budget support; plan for and allocate resources to get the most for the money; and engage in fund-raising and entrepreneurial activities. Furthermore, librarians must be aware of global economic trends that may affect the business of library management and carefully monitor trends in the climate in which the library operates. This involves scanning or reading professional literature in library and information science, information technology, and the health care management fields as well as networking with colleagues inside the profession and within the institution in which one works.

This chapter provides an overview of processes involved in responsible fiscal management with one caveat: no chapter can replace the need for each librarian to keep up with what is happening in one's own institution and the health care economy overall because these factors control the fate of the library. The reader will want to refer to Chapter 4, Marketing Library Services, for ideas for combining fiscal management with techniques in marketing programs and strengthening the credibility of the library.

BUDGETING AND FISCAL MANAGEMENT TECHNIQUES

Prentice states that

> financial planning for library and information services is carried out in a complex environment. Past and present trends outside the library affect budget planning as much or more than any internal cost analyses or dollar figures [2].

Having a strategic plan for the future of the library is the required first step to preparing a budget. Planned expenditures should flow from a well-articulated set of long-term goals and objectives. Defining the role of the library over the coming years is imperative so that purchases can be made when needed and the appropriate programs are available at the opportune time.

After appropriate planning for services, one of a manager's primary responsibilities is to secure the resources needed to carry out the mission and program of the library. Success in budgeting determines success in other areas [3], because the budget brings to fruition both the short-term and longer-range plans for the library. The budget links programs, services, and activities that have been articulated during the planning process and validated by those with whom the library works: administrators, library users, the library advisory committee, and staff members. A good budget assists in evaluation of the library's plan and is used as a monitoring tool for library activities. A library manager can expect to be held accountable for budget preparation, management, and review and is often evaluated based on success in this area.

Budgeting represents an active, year-round process, and Rounds [4] identifies the following steps in budget development:

1. Plan and identify needs.
2. Analyze and prioritize activities and services.
3. Identify revenues and expenditures.
4. Develop initial budget.
5. Evaluate initial budget.
6. Develop budget.
7. Develop budget presentation.
8. Present budget.
9. Redevelop budget.

10. Obtain budget approval.
11. Implement budget.
12. Manage budget.

To improve communication and fiscal monitoring, the library administrator may wish to develop a budget calendar that includes various dates associated with specific activities [5]. Although most operating budgets work on an annual cycle, some institutions use two-year cycles. In either case, the more time available to gather information, the better the presentation, and a calendar enables the manager to have a sense of what needs to be done at all times throughout the year.

Many types of budgets are possible, and the type of budget prepared by the library manager will be dictated by the institution. Usually a budget packet of some sort will be received that contains instructions on budget preparation, relevant forms to complete, a timetable with due dates, and other appropriate information. It is important to have data to document the budget request, especially since library expenses rarely go down and often increase at a rate higher than the general inflationary rate on consumer prices. Some institutions require estimates of expenditures by month, and libraries need to make clear that disproportionate expenditures will occur in the month that journal subscriptions or other large expenses will be paid. Some institutions make special funds available outside the normal budget process or will provide the opportunity for departments to submit requests for budget supplements. In all cases, familiarity with institutional budgetary and funding processes is imperative to receiving support for library programs.

Traditional budget types include lump sum, line item, formula, program, performance and zero based, all of which have been well described by Braude, Warner, and others [6-7]. A brief description of each of these budget types follows.

With a *lump sum budget,* the library receives an allocation of a set amount of money to cover all expenses for a fiscal cycle. The library manager determines how funds will be spent. While this allows considerable flexibility, it often complicates the task of relating the budget to the goals of the library and justifying the need for increases in expenditures in specific areas where costs tend to increase substantially and regularly.

In a *line item budget,* the institution defines specific categories, each with a line that indicates the maximum amount to be spent on that area. Examples include salaries; library materials such as books, journals, audiovisuals, and databases; contracted services; or general operating expenses. A line item budget allows individual categories of expenditures to be justified separately and requires careful monitoring throughout the year to be sure that expenses are charged to the appropriate line. Some institutions require line budgeting, then allow flexibility in shifting funds across lines while others mandate staying within the budget for each category. Institutions that allow movement across lines will often require special approval for salary adjustments or establishment of additional personnel positions even when uncommitted funds are available in other budget lines.

Formula budgets are most often used in public or university libraries where funds are allocated based on factors such as number of students in a specific program, user population, or geographic area served in the case of public libraries. As the relationships between teaching hospitals and medical schools change and health systems expand, formula budgets may become more popular when libraries negotiate agreements to provide services to institutions other than their parent. Fees may then be based on the number of physicians and other health professionals to whom services will be offered.

A *program budget* focuses on what the library does for people and measures library programs against the goals of the organization the library serves. For example, the cost of a library's educational program can be described and budgeted separately from that of its reference service. Essentially, a line budget is prepared for each program the library offers. This type of budget is useful as new programs are proposed since they need to be carefully costed out prior to implementation. Difficulties with this type of budget arise when one program is funded and another is deleted yet personnel are split among the programs. For example, a full-time librarian may teach, provide reference services, and do Web development, spending one-third time on each activity. If one program is eliminated, how is that third of the salary then covered? In such a case, the library administrator must find alternate funds to cover one-third of the personnel costs.

A *performance budget* appears similar to a program budget in that it requires both determining individual programs and calculating their costs. It involves identifying how individuals spend their time and allocating those costs over the programs on which they are working. It enables determination of unit costs for activities, such as the cost to catalog a book or answer a reference question.

Zero-based budgeting involves determining what should happen in the library in the next year and projecting the cost for each activity. Theoretically, it ignores what has happened in the past or what is happening now. Each proposed activity is called a "decision package," and a list of questions must be addressed for each "package." Questions include the name of the program, steps required to carry it out, who will benefit, consequences of having no program, alternative ways to perform the work, the proposed budget, and a priority rank for this program vis-à-vis all the programs in the library proposal.

Recently a number of academic medical centers have adopted the practice of responsibility-centered management, which has been described as a process that shares resource allocation decisions through a partnership among academic faculty, support units, and central administration [8]. Under this model, both the allocation and generation of revenues become shared responsibilities, and budget preparation takes into account all expenses including those for things such as space and all revenue, including that for overhead on grants and income from endowment funds. Responsibility-centered management carries enormous budget and effort implications for libraries in institutions where this takes place. Libraries may need to negotiate receiving funds from each unit/department on campus to which it provides services rather than with one central administration or dean of a specific school.

The library and other service units will come under increasing scrutiny under responsibility-centered management, and they will experience enormous pressure to demonstrate the value of services provided. Yet, in more enlightened implementations, benefits may ensue because careful consideration may be given to core interdisciplinary activities such as libraries, and efforts are made to ensure adequate financing for central support services. On the other hand, one danger is that smaller, departmentally based libraries can appear to be more responsive to user needs and able to provide special services to the revenue center that cannot be provided by a centralized library entity. This perception can weaken the support for the central library.

Besides these common techniques, other budgeting methods exist. There is no "right" way to do a budget. In preparing a budget, it is imperative that the library manager be familiar with institutional policies and procedures as well as rules and regulations. While the budget must meet institutional requirements, it can also serve as a tool for planning and articulating library programs and should be viewed as a vital opportunity to garner essential funds for the library.

COSTING OF SERVICES

Snyder and Davenport remind us that "one of the primary reasons for gathering and analyzing cost information is to assist management in planning and controlling the operations of an organization" [9]. Knowing the cost of services enables the librarian to make better informed decisions, to consciously determine when a service may no longer be viable, to prepare a cost/benefit analysis, and to establish a fee schedule if costs are to be assessed. Accountants establish activity-based cost systems as an accounting information system that focuses on the underlying activities necessary to produce a product or provide a service [10]. In preparing to determine the cost of a library service, it is necessary to understand the concepts of direct and indirect costs. *Direct costs* are those that can be traced to a particular cost objective, anything within the organization whose costs need to be measured, such as running a reference service. *Indirect costs*, sometimes called *overhead,* are cost objectives that cannot be tied to one particular service—for example, the utilities or administrative costs of running a library [11].

Understanding the difference between *fixed* and *variable costs* is essential prior to analyzing a service cost. A cost is fixed if it remains unchanged despite fluctuations in activity level. An example is the cost to license a database or electronic journal for an unlimited amount of use by everyone in the institution. Variable costs change directly in proportion to activity. For instance, when an online system vendor charges by the connect hour, the longer it takes to search a database and the more citations retrieved, the higher the cost. The addition of Internet access in libraries has changed fixed and variable costs for telecommunications. Prior to the Internet, many libraries had recurring variable costs for communicating with service providers for cataloging and database access via standard telephone lines. Once access to these services became available over the Internet, a flat communication access rate became possible, although there may still be variations in monthly cost based on number of items retrieved or records updated.

Why are these concepts important? Increasingly health care organizations are being asked to analyze and explain their costs to the public, elected officials, government agencies, managed care organizations, and insurers. As health care costs become more carefully scrutinized, every expenditure is reviewed and libraries must be able to explain and justify their costs. Furthermore, as hospitals that formerly were closely integrated with academic institutions are being reorganized, merged, or sold to for-profit organizations, libraries will need to contribute data to the process of negotiating for payment for services shared by the hospital and the academic center. In time, one library might be asked to provide service to five hospitals that become members of the same health system. Or, that one library might be asked to provide services to multiple discrete institutions on a contractual basis. Hence, it is important to know how to calculate the full cost of providing a service. For example, if databases and full-text journals are to be available on hospital workstations and the hospital is to pay the library to provide that access, the library administrator must identify all costs and decide which ones to include in its charges to the hospital.

The ability to determine costs has become more complicated as technology has been thoroughly integrated into services that health sciences libraries provide. Today, computer-based catalogs enable us to know what resources are available, online access to databases has replaced use of printed indexes as the most common means of identifying information, users expect journals to be available electronically as well as in print form, and students learn from computer-based educational programs in addition to studying textbooks. However, whereas most paper-based resources had long life cycles and could be viewed as onetime expenditures, computer-based systems need frequent updating and replacement. With a card catalog, new cards were added, outdated records removed, and new drawers occasionally purchased. With online systems, the computer housing the database and software needs to be upgraded regularly, and usually an annual maintenance fee must be paid to the vendor who provides the system. One management strategy to deal with these recurring costs is to develop a regular replacement schedule for computer equipment, knowing that everything needs to be replaced on a two-, three-, or four-year cycle. This point is not to imply that computer-based systems do not provide added value but to advise that they do change the factors involved in costing out a service.

Automation further complicates cost analysis because systems often support multiple services. For instance, the online catalog may function as the front-end interface to other databases and electronic resources licensed by the library. One may or may not wish to allocate some of the online catalog costs to the category of end user searching, and it may be difficult to determine an amount for this allocation. At the same time, computers can be a major asset in helping libraries track and analyze costs. Many commercial accounting software packages are available to libraries. Alternatively, most libraries use database software to track their expenditures in a line item budget or by cost center when funds are coming from multiple sources. Having these data readily available makes it much easier to determine how funds are being spent and to answer questions that arise when analyzing the types of costs previously described.

A related issue is the need to budget for more *capital expenditures* in an automated environment. While institutional definitions of capital vary, most include a minimum base dollar amount and a minimal life expectancy. For example, any item costing $500 or more with a useful life of at least one year might be considered a capital item. Thus, in addition to being costly, computers, computer systems, and peripherals almost always fall under the rules for capital rather than recurring expenditures. Sometimes capital allocation is done outside the regular budget process even if capital requests are submitted as part of the regular budget package.

ACCESS VERSUS OWNERSHIP

Even a library that has excellent data and can identify and justify all its expenditures must take care to explain why the cost of operating the library continues to increase faster than the general rate of inflation as calculated by the U.S. Consumer Price Index. The biggest culprit remains the cost of serial publications that continues as the largest category of expenditure after personnel in most health sciences libraries. Brandon and Hill report a 24% increase in the price of serials included on their selected list of books and journals for the small medical library between 1995 and 1997 [12]. Alexander and Dingley show medical journals, with a $524.65 average price, as the third most expensive subject category in their 1998 U.S. periodical price study. Medicine ranks second in the percentage of price increase, with an average annual jump of 13.7%, between 1996-97 and 1997-98 [13]. EBSCO Subscription Services, in its annual Index Medicus Price Study, clearly and graphically provides information on inflationary trends over the past five years and provides data to assist librarians in making informed budgetary arguments and decisions [14].

From a financial planning point of view, it is necessary to look at the cumulative cost of acquiring and owning materials before they are requested versus the cost of purchasing an item on demand. Today, more than ever, it is not possible for every library to own all items or resources that every patron needs to complete his or her work. So, how does one determine when to buy an item now in case someone needs it tomorrow or when to wait to purchase that item at the time it is specifically requested? Since journals still account for the bulk of library materials expenditures, one simple formula to assess the value of a serial is to divide the serial subscription cost by the number of documented uses. This provides a cost-per-use value that can be used in determining whether it is more cost-effective to subscribe to a journal or purchase individual articles when needed. From a financial planning point of view, it is necessary to look at all the costs of owning materials compared to the cost to purchase an item on demand. In the case of journal ownership, one must factor in more than just the initial subscription price. Costs also include such items as the cost of housing material, providing it to users, binding, providing equipment for an audiovisual or electronic supplements, cataloging, and other factors as appropriate for the item in question.

In determining an access cost, on the other hand, price calculations must include such expenses as rush order charges or providing staff to locate an item, purchase or borrow that item, and then return or reshelve the item if appropriate. Again, this is not a comprehensive list of factors but a sample of financial issues to be considered when determining the best way to make materials available within the constraints of a limited budget.

Health sciences libraries have also chosen to stretch scarce dollars by banding together in consortia to provide access to additional resources. Through its National Network of Libraries of Medicine, the National Library of Medicine provides a structure both for interlibrary loan among libraries and for providing documents directly to individuals. Organizations such as OhioLINK enable broad, statewide access to academic library resources for students and faculty no matter where they live or work. The Medical Library Center of New York consortium includes both a storage facility and a shared collection of journals for use by members and others. Libraries in newly merged health systems are cooperating and increasing availability of electronic resources by jointly licensing access to materials as a way to deal with high prices.

Determining whether to provide materials just in case or enable access only when needed is an issue that will receive increasing attention in libraries as it has in other areas of business. The American Society for Information Science's 1994 annual meeting focused on issues related to the economics of information, and several of the papers in the proceedings are relevant to this discussion [15]. For further information on budgeting for collections, see Volume 4 in this series, *Collection Development and Assessment in Health Sciences Libraries.*

LICENSING AND CONTRACTING FOR SERVICES

Throughout history, health sciences libraries have purchased materials for their collections. With the advent of substantial content in electronic format, publishers may now license material—databases, serials, and books—rather than making it available for sale. This is a rapidly changing area, with each publisher setting independent policies. When librarians find themselves negotiating an ongoing license instead of purchasing an item one time, the financial implications of licensing need to be carefully reviewed, especially as computer software becomes sophisticated enough to enable a per-use charge. Electronic services share several characteristics: they will probably require continuing annual payments, and they do not belong to the library but are leased for the period for which payment has been received [16]. The Association of Research Libraries (ARL), the Medical Library Association (MLA), and other professional associations have developed principles for negotiating licenses. The ARL Web site is a good place to check for the latest information in this area: http://arl.cni.org/scomm/licensing.

The library manager must also consider the financial impact of licensing electronic access to materials that often duplicate print sources that have already been purchased. It is not feasible over the long term to pay for information twice, yet many publishers bundle print and nonprint costs or only allow electronic access to a journal in conjunction with a print subscription. Collection development considerations have to be weighed against financial considerations, the dynamic nature of technological progress, and user demands.

For many years, hospital libraries have been contracting for services such as cataloging. Smaller libraries often find it more cost effective to pay an outside service to provide cataloging data, either in card or electronic format, than to hire the extra staff necessary to catalog a small number of items inhouse. An extension of this approach is to contract with a vendor, another library, or a consortium to provide an online catalog and related components. Some libraries include serials check-in service as a part of the contracted service. In arranging for contracted services, the manager should obtain a written agreement that clearly specifies the services to be provided, the cost of the services, performance expectations, and the method of dispute resolution should problems arise. This agreement should include a clause specifying notification requirements for nonrenewal and may specify a penalty should the work not be completed. Institutional policy will determine whether an attorney reviews all contracts for service, but the library administrator must often understand basic elements of contract law.

This combination of legal and fiscal knowledge comes into play in many ways. For example, librarians are increasingly considering leasing rather than purchasing services. A lease may allow the library to provide service to its patrons in a more cost-effective manner. With the use of multiyear and fixed-lease payments, it might be possible to temporarily hold costs in check at a time when inflation would normally increase the cost of operations [17]. To evaluate a lease from a financial viewpoint, current costs of operations must be analyzed and compared with lease costs to determine savings or other advantages. If the choice is made to lease, performance standards must be outlined, then compared to actual performance once the contract is in place. Leasing can be especially effective in dealing with expensive equipment that has a finite life expectancy, such as photocopiers and computers.

LIBRARY DEVELOPMENT AND FUND-RAISING

In the 1990s, the economics of health care occupies national attention, and Dalrymple believes that this decade will be characterized by too much information and too few resources [18]. To combat the demand for expanded services without increased institutionally budgeted funds, libraries have devoted increased attention to identifying external resources to support new programs, facilities, technologies, and services. Consequently, position descriptions for library directors have come to include fund-raising experience as another skill required for the job. The successful library administrator will devise strategies to tap external funds from a variety of potential sources.

Library development programs derive from the culture of the institution in which they exist. It is both important and necessary to understand whether the parent institution demands that all fund-raising be carried out by a central development office working in partnership with units such as the library. Alternatively, it may be acceptable for units to raise funds in a decentralized manner, going directly to agencies or individuals to seek contributions. In both cases, it is incumbent on the library manager to have at his or her fingertips a list of ideas for program enhancements and their associated costs should the opportunity arise to make a case for outside funds.

A 1992 survey of members of the Association of Research Libraries found that fund-raising in these libraries is well developed [19]. Numerous ARL ideas may be useful to health sciences libraries, such as how to

- participate in general fund-raising activities taking place in the parent institution;
- devote budgetary funds to a dedicated library development program;
- fund-raise for a specific program, such as the library collection, automation, preservation, or building renovation;
- negotiate for a major gift from a donor or foundation;
- develop a capital campaign for the library;
- organize an annual fund-raising activity;
- work with a friends of the library group; and
- prepare case statements for specific fund-raising efforts.

Involvement in fund-raising presents many questions:

- Will dollars raised by libraries result in reduced budgetary allocations from the institution's administration?
- How can libraries identify prospects for the library's development program, and should these be coordinated with similar activities in the institution?
- Do libraries have or should libraries devote resources and staffing to development efforts?
- Are library friends groups effective, and should they confine themselves to library-wide fund-raising or devote themselves to special projects [20]?

Each library must weigh the pros and cons of engaging in active development campaigns and become aware of institutional policies and prohibitions in dealing with donors. The concepts of fund-raising may seem foreign to many health sciences librarians, but donors make money available to librarians who are willing and able to devote time and effort to researching and implementing fund-raising programs. Successful fund-raising flows from effective planning: What is the current status of the library? What is it becoming? What does the library need to get there? Answering these questions before fund-raising begins is an important part of the process [21-22].

Funds also may come from outside sources such as foundations or government granting agencies. An institutional grants and contracts office may provide information and assistance in identifying and applying to these programs. Individuals within an institution may have a special interest in the medical library. The development office of the organization may offer guidelines in approaching these sources. In any case, the fund-raiser matches a project within the library with a potential grantor's goals. The project identified may not be one that will solve the library's most pressing problem, but it may allow the library to add equipment or a service that would not otherwise be possible.

The National Library of Medicine (NLM) supports several grant programs for medical libraries that it updates to reflect what it views as important programmatic areas. Examples from the 1990s include providing funds to assist libraries to gain Internet access and enhancing effective use of computer and telecommunications technology in the delivery of health information to underserved practitioner populations. Information on NLM grant programs is available from the library, through the National Network of Libraries of Medicine, and at the NLM Web site.

Foundations may also be a source for grants to health sciences libraries. Obtaining private funding is a time intensive project that involves considerable collaboration with institutional development offices and research into what a particular foundation may fund. Different groups support different types of projects, specialize in certain service areas, or limit their interest to a geographic area. Some foundations will not pay for building projects; others will not support publications or endowments; most will not provide money for day-to-day operations. Increasingly, matching funds are required to show that either the institutional support for the project or other external support exists. The publications of the Foundation Center are useful in researching outside funding, in particular *The Foundation Directory* [23]. In addition to maintaining the Foundation Center headquarters in New York City, the organization places resources on deposit in public and other types of libraries throughout the United States.

Preparing a proposal for a funding agency, whether a government agency or a private foundation, requires gathering information on the type of projects previously funded and paying close attention to the instructions for preparing and submitting the proposal. Often there are specific forms to complete, signatures to obtain, commitments to make regarding the period after initial support is provided, and requirements regarding cost sharing. Many funding organizations employ grant officers who can be quite helpful in explaining their policies, procedures, and time lines. Submitting proposals that do not fit the agency's focus wastes both the librarian's time and the funding agency's resources.

Sometimes in the proposal review process the agency makes a site visit to a library that requests funding. To prepare, the librarian should find out what is to be accomplished during the visit and negotiate a schedule for the visit. Individuals who are to attend should be identified and scheduled. The librarian should involve key people within the institution to demonstrate the importance of the project, even if the site visitors did not request their presence. The names and institutional affiliations of the site visitors should be requested to research their background and interests prior to their arrival.

Meeting accommodations should be finalized well in advance. If a tour is part of the visit, everyone in the institution, and particularly the staff whose areas might be visited, should know who is visiting along with the reason for and importance of the visit.

In some cases, a mock site visit proves useful. Small items make a good impression, such as advising people to wear identification badges and preparing nametags for the visitors, arranging for refreshments, and cleaning the facility. Efforts should be made to adhere to the schedule, but the institution should also be prepared for changes in the schedule or to answer questions asked by the visitors even if they seem somewhat peripheral to the project for which funding has been requested. Upon completion of the visit, a written thank-you note should be sent to the agency or foundation along with responses to any questions that remained unanswered during the visit.

In another approach to fund-raising, the librarian pursues support for programs either through a formally organized friends of the library group or by approaching an already existing group, such as an alumni association or medical or auxiliary board. An advantage to the latter is that the library may apply directly to a group with a preexisting awareness of the library and an assumed interest in maintaining a high-quality information resource. Also, the library does not have to build and administratively sustain a specialized friends organization.

If funding from such existing institutional groups is not possible, it may be worth weighing the benefits and drawbacks of a friends organization. Little has been written about friends groups in medical libraries, although some do exist and make real contributions to the libraries they support [24-25]. Aside from the financial assistance provided by a friends group, the higher level of visibility and support that a friends group offers has real value. The primary drawback of a friends organization is the amount of personnel time spent in organizing and supporting such a group. Initial costs for printing and secretarial support also need to be met. Sometimes, when the costs in time and money of maintaining a friends group are factored in, it becomes clear that the nonfinancial advantages are the primary benefit.

Friends groups often provide funding for needs that may have limited appeal to outside sources. Friends groups may provide endowment funds; support for a specific collection or program, such as archives, special collections, or electronic resources; or the matching funds needed to comply with a foundation grant. Individual friends can also identify prospects for future larger gifts or provide contacts with potential donors who might not otherwise be familiar with the library program. Yet, numerous operational questions are associated with establishing a friends organization:

- Who would join this group?
- What benefits would they receive for joining?

- What programs or services might be expected by members?
- How, specifically, will the library benefit from the friends [26]?

Other important questions to answer relating to the establishment of a friends group include these:

- Who will provide administrative support for the friends, both the initial and the ongoing support?
- What will be the library director's role vis-à-vis the friends group?
- Who will pay the administrative costs of operating a friends group?
- Who are the natural leaders of the group and how can the library help them step forward?
- Will there be regular meetings?
- Will the cost of sustaining such a group exceed income or intangible benefits?

Many articles and resources are available to help librarians research, implement, and sustain a friends group [27-28]. In addition, the Friends of Libraries U.S.A. (FOLUSA), based in Philadelphia, publishes monographs, directories, newsletters, and fact sheets about all aspects of friends groups. While not aimed specifically at medical libraries, they do provide useful information to academic and smaller libraries [29].

Raising funds for the library also occurs through development of partnerships or the formation of alliances. Mielke calls corporate partnerships a practical approach to managing the library in an era when library services are not fully funded [30]. Berman, however, cautions against "selling our souls and becoming like shills for enterprises that frequently are more concerned about marketing their wares than in really promoting literacy, democracy, or self-empowerment" [31]. Medical libraries, like other types of libraries, must weigh the boon of a corporate partner sponsoring a service that might not otherwise be provided against possible partisanship reflected in documents or publicity for the program. Should a database vendor sponsor a library Web page that includes links to that vendor's product? Or should a fast-food restaurant logo appear on the library's guide to sources of nutrition information? In an era when patrons are familiar with seeing logos everywhere, the library manager must balance the advantages and disadvantages of corporate partnership.

Another opportunity for libraries to raise revenue exists through establishing fee-based services to be offered to the public, to other types of libraries, and to small businesses that do not have their own library services. Services that can be offered for a fee typically include research, reference, educational programs, and document delivery. However, prior to establishing the service, a thorough cost analysis must be completed both to ensure that it is worthwhile to the library to offer the service and to establish appropriate pricing. For further information on budgeting for fee-based services, see volume 3 in this series, *Information Access and Delivery in Health Sciences Libraries.*

Library managers have a paramount responsibility to engage in sound fiscal management. They need to know the policies and procedures of their parent institution and how to prepare a budget that both presents the library program and conforms to local regulations. The cost of services should be clearly articulated and easily explained. The administrator must consider carefully decisions regarding performing services locally, contracting with others to provide the service, or acting as a service provider. Opportunities to seek outside funds should be pursued and entrepreneurial activities identified, keeping within the mission of the library and institution. The more and better information the library manager obtains and creates, the greater the likelihood the manager will be respected for leadership in administering successful and well-funded programs. Experienced library administrators view fiscal management as both a fundamental responsibility and an essential tool.

REFERENCES

1. Mahar, M. Tomorrow's hospital: for profit or not, it will be radically different. Barron's 1994 Jan;72(4):12-18.

2. Prentice A. Financial planning for libraries. 2nd ed. Lanham, MD: Scarecrow Press, 1996:1. (The library administration no. 8)

3. Braude RM. Administration: general principles applied to health science libraries. In: Darling L, Colaianni LA, Bishop D, eds. Handbook of medical library practice. 4th ed. v. 3. Chicago: Medical Library Association, 1988:221-85.

4. Rounds RS. Basic budget practices for librarians. 2nd ed. Chicago: American Library Association, 1994:6.

5. Hill MK. Budget and financial record keeping in the small library. 2nd ed. Chicago: Library Administration and Management Association, American Library Association, 1993:2.

6. Braude, op. cit., 259.

7. Warner AS. Owning your numbers: an introduction to budgeting for special libraries. Washington, DC: Special Libraries Association, 1992:13-19.

8. Whalen EL. Responsibility centered budgeting: an approach for institutions of higher education. Bloomington: Indiana University Press, 1991.

9. Snyder H, Davenport E. Costing and pricing in the digital age: a practical guide for information services. New York: Neal-Schuman, 1997:10.

10. Livingstone JL. The portable MBA in finance and accounting. New York: Wiley, 1992.

11. Snyder, op. cit.

12. Brandon AN, Hill DR. Selected list of books and journals for the small medical library. Bull Med Libr Assoc 1997;85(2):111-35.

34 Administration and Management

13. Alexander AW, Dingley B. U.S. periodical prices 1998. American Libraries 1998;29(5):82-90.

14. Fortney LM, Basile VA. Index Medicus price study 1993-1997. Birmingham, AL: EBSCO Subscription Services, 1998.

15. Maxian B. The economics of information: proceedings of the 57th ASIS Annual Meeting. Silver Springs, MD: American Society for Information Science, 1994.

16. Martin MS. Collection development and finance: a guide to strategic library materials budgeting. Chicago: American Library Association, 1995.

17. Smith GS. Managerial accounting for libraries and other non-profit organizations. Chicago: American Library Association, 1991.

18. Dalrymple PW. Introduction. Libr Trends 1993 Sum;42(1):1-4.

19. Claassen LC. Library development and fundraising. Washington, DC: Association of Research Libraries, 1993. (Association of Research Libraries SPEC Kit 193)

20. Ibid.

21. Steele V, Elder SD. Becoming a fundraiser: the principles and practice of library development. Chicago: American Library Association, 1992.

22. Barber P. Getting your grant: a how-to manual for librarians. New York: Neal-Schuman, 1993.

23. Tuller M. The foundation directory. New York: Foundation Center, 1998.

24. Mueller MH, Overmeier J. An examination of characteristics related to success of friends groups in medical school rare book libraries. Bull Med Libr Assoc 1981 Jan;69(1):9-13.

25. Leatherbury MC, Lyders RA. Friends of library groups in health sciences libraries. Bull Med Libr Assoc 1978 Jul;66(3):315-8.

26. Corson-Finnerty A, Blanchard L. Using the Web to find old friends and e-friends. Amer Libr 1998;29(4):90-91.

27. Hood JM. Fundraising for nonprofit institutions. Greenwich, CT: JAI Press, 1987.

28. Krummel DW. Organizing the library's support: donors, volunteers, friends. Urbana: University of Illinois Graduate School of Library Science, 1980.

29. Dolnick S. Friends of libraries sourcebook. 3rd ed. Chicago: American Library Association, 1990.

30. Mielke L, Berman S. What price partnerships? Amer Libr 1998;29(2):43-6.

31. Ibid.

3

Human Resources Management

Carol Jenkins

Health sciences libraries and librarians are experiencing dramatic changes in response to changes in information technology and the health care industry and academic environments in which they operate. In this new era, librarians have taken on expanded roles in managing information technology as well as integrating and managing the full range of mission-critical information for their organizations. Librarians work with other information professionals and library support staff to function as knowledge workers who create, integrate, and manage access to information in all its forms. Studies have shown that the knowledge, skills, and abilities most needed by health sciences library workers today include flexibility, adaptability, and risk acceptance in addition to analytical, organizational, technical, and other skills. As service organizations, libraries must view the staff as their most valuable asset. As the roles of health sciences libraries change to meet the needs of their clientele, it is vital that the library administrator maximize the value of the library staff within the parent organization. In today's rapidly changing environment, achieving the maximum contribution by the staff requires careful attention to all aspects of the human resources management process.

This chapter will touch on the basic components of human resources management: what it takes to attract, recruit, hire, enable, evaluate, reward, develop, and deploy the best possible library staff. These embody the central elements of a human resources system. They should relate closely to one another and to the library's overall priorities. Even though most library directors work in organizations that maintain their own human resources offices and set some policies and practices applicable to all employees, it is important to understand the basic human resources processes and functions in order to interpret and apply them in the best interests of the library and its staff.

THE CHANGING HEALTH CARE
AND INFORMATION ENVIRONMENT

The landmark Matheson Report noted in 1982 that "few organizations are as information-dependent as the academic health sciences center (AHSC) and few professions are as information-intensive as medicine" [1]. Today's health care environment, characterized by increased competition, rapid technological change, and the development of multiple health care delivery systems, depends on information more than ever before [2]. The health care industry is becoming multisystem, creating more interdependence of previously separate entities [3]. One key element of such systems is their reliance on sharing information about all aspects of the health care delivery process. The very nature of work performed in this environment has also changed. Zuboff has coined the phrase "the informated environment" [4]. In this environment, she claims, the worker has access to information about the whole system of activities to which the work is related and is called upon to make different, often more complex, kinds of decisions as a result.

Furthermore, information technology has greatly expanded access to health care information for consumers as well as for health care workers. Health care consumers demand better information, greater access to health information, and integral involvement in their own and their families' health care decisions. Health care reform efforts place a high value on cost-effective care for all, with access to relevant information being a cornerstone for determining both the cost and the quality of care.

The rapid expansion of published information in the sciences, its high cost, and opportunities for electronic publishing push libraries into a new information environment. Braude calls attention to the impact of information technology on the traditional roles of health sciences librarians. He notes that "new forms of information appear almost daily" and that librarians are not well represented among researchers engaged in the development and application of these new forms because they have been trained to deal with the container rather than the content of information [5]. Traditional library services also have evolved or been transformed by technology and changing user needs.

THE CHANGING HEALTH SCIENCES LIBRARIAN

The health sciences librarian must understand the changing aspects of the information process and must possess the skills to support that process.

Matheson cites the need for "a significant talent pool in the area of health information and library sciences," noting that "the appropriate professional skills . . . must be continually developed" [6]. Many reports in the past decade have affirmed that the role of the library and the librarian are indeed changing and that new knowledge and skills will be required to address those changes [7-11]. While strong voices predict that the profession will not adapt well enough to changing needs, Lucier, Molholt, and others present compelling visions in which successful health sciences libraries and librarians are prominent [12-13]. The Medical Library Association (MLA) has recognized the need to redefine the role of the health sciences librarian in the new information environment. Its publication *Value of the Hospital Library* discusses the impact of library services on patient care and the value of the library for hospital administrators and staff [14].

In her Janet Doe Lecture at the 1989 Medical Library Association Annual Meeting, Anderson asserts that "the library resource most critical to achievement . . . is the caliber and qualities of the people, the librarians" [15]. Reviewing the qualities, educational backgrounds, and societal influences that have shaped the recruitment of professional medical librarians over the past century, she calls attention to the attributes typically valued in librarians, including some "double-edged swords." For example, a strong personal service orientation is highly valued, but, all too often, someone else derives the complete credit for publications that rely on work done largely by the librarian.

New attributes are valued in today's health sciences librarian, according to Anderson [16]:

- *Technical literacy:* being conversant with information technology and knowledgeable about database design and function
- *Research competence:* entailing, at minimum, familiarity with research methods; it is increasingly important for librarians to conduct research to determine user information behavior and needs and to use the results to improve services
- *Service orientation:* deriving assertive, client-centered programs driven by acknowledged technical expertise and subject background
- *Management abilities:* attaining proficiencies in interpersonal relations and external communications
- *Leadership qualities:* exerting leadership not only among other librarians but within the broader organizational context, thus positioning the library as an effective player in the overall administrative and planning framework of the institution
- *Knowledge of the organization:* understanding one's environmental context and the functional role of information within it; as libraries become intricately intertwined with more units outside familiar domains, political savvy is critical for negotiating and building coalitions

Building on these attributes, MLA has outlined core areas of knowledge for health sciences librarianship. Demonstration of continued competence is required for admission to MLA's Academy of Health Information Professionals. These areas of knowledge also serve as a basis for *Platform for Change*, MLA's 1991 educational policy statement. This statement acknowledges the pivotal role of the health sciences librarian in the handling of biomedical information. It offers recommendations for individuals, organizations, and institutions to provide the learning opportunities needed by librarians if they are to keep pace with rapid, continuous change. The MLA process that identified the core areas of knowledge is described by Roper and Mayfield [17].

The core areas of knowledge described in *Platform for Change* are as follows [18]:

- *Health sciences environment and information policies:* understanding the contexts in which biomedical information needs occur
- *Management of information service:* acquiring skills in applying the principles of library and information science to a health sciences environment
- *Health sciences information services:* gaining knowledge of the content of health-related information resources and skills in using them
- *Health sciences resource management:* mastering theory and demonstrating skill in identifying, collecting, evaluating, and organizing resources and developing and providing databases
- *Information systems and technology:* understanding the continuum ranging from basic automation principles to shaping information systems that meet institutional needs
- *Instructional support system:* holding knowledge of learning theory and its application in teaching how to access, organize, and use information to solve health-related problems
- *Research, analysis, and interpretation:* understanding the theoretical basis of information and knowledge management and applying it to conduct and interpret research

Bowden and Olivier conducted a survey of medical librarian employers in 1988, and a follow-up survey in 1992, to learn more about what employers expect of entry-level librarians [19]. They report that the skills valued most highly by employers in 1992 included problem-solving and analytical skills, microcomputer skills, bibliographic instruction, online searching, reference/information service, and MEDLINE searching skills. The qualities most highly sought included communication skills, enthusiasm, self-esteem, flexibility, service orientation, willingness to be a team player, and interpersonal skills. Intellectual curiosity, professional attitude, and leadership potential were also highly valued. However, respondents to both surveys reported difficulties in attracting applicants with these skills and attributes. The small size of applicant pools was a common concern.

Anderson concludes that if the library profession wants to compete effectively for the best people in today's market, which places a high premium on the information and knowledge worker, it must reexamine the qualities and abilities that it has traditionally sought. The profession must question whether the current workforce possesses the skills and attitudes required for today and tomorrow. Employers must seek individuals who demonstrate the best of the aforementioned attributes, as well as competency in the core areas of knowledge. To attract strong candidates for library openings, librarians must be seen as the information leaders within their organizations. Employers must define exciting job opportunities and reward staff appropriately. For further discussion of how libraries and librarians can adapt to changing roles, see *Symposium: Platform for Change: Medical Library Education in the Information Age* [20].

What implications does this hold for the library director or administrator who wants to recruit and retain the best-qualified health sciences library staff? Job announcements for professional librarians today may call for familiarity with a variety of electronic information systems and services, advanced subject knowledge in a health or science discipline, teaching skills, research and evaluation expertise, and excellent communication skills, in addition to the graduate library degree. One recent job advertisement from an academic health sciences library seeks an individual with "leadership accomplishments in redefining programs, implementing new services, setting strategic directions, and fostering partnerships" as well as the "ability to lead a diverse staff in a rapidly changing, technology-intense environment; to work effectively and collaboratively in a complex organization; and to engender a flexible and supportive work environment" [21]. Depending on how the library defines its role in knowledge management, some directors may recruit experts whose professional training is in a health discipline, rather than in librarianship. Library support staff with a broader variety of skills and mastery of more complex skills will also be needed. These skills may include expertise with electronic information systems, telecommunications, or supervision and management and the ability to work in teams to create and provide products and services.

The health sciences library staff work in organizations that are abandoning traditional hierarchical arrangements in favor of group structures that use cross-functional planning and coordination of activities [22]. These new approaches offer staff at all levels of the organization challenging opportunities to contribute their ideas and expertise, and they also allow staff to participate in decision making in more ways. They require a staff whose knowledge and abilities are up-to-date and conducive to teamwork and a library director who is committed to the development of staff as the library's most critical resource.

MLA's *Platform for Change* emphasizes the importance of both the individual's and the employer's responsibility for professional development for health sciences librarians in response to evolving roles [23]. Following the publication of MLA's educational policy statement, in 1995 the National Library of Medicine (NLM) issued its *Long-Range Plan on the Education and Training of Health Sciences Librarians.* This report outlines key responsibilities at the individual, institutional, and national levels for assuring that health sciences librarians gain the knowledge and skills they need throughout their careers [24]. As a result of this plan, NLM awarded planning grants to a number of health sciences libraries and library schools to develop new educational models and programs aimed at health sciences information professionals [25].

THE HUMAN RESOURCES FUNCTION

According to Creth and Duda, the human resources function in a library exists to help ensure that the needs of the organization and its individual staff are met appropriately [26]. Human resources support is provided in health sciences libraries through various means. Only the largest libraries will be able to support a position dedicated to this function. Others turn to human resources professionals in their parent institutions or hospitals for assistance with recruitment, compensation, position classification, counseling, legal issues, training and development, and the like. Effective support in the aforementioned areas is critical for optimum staff recruitment, effectiveness, and staff satisfaction. Library administrators stand to gain multiple benefits from cultivating a close collaborative relationship with the central human resources unit in their organizations, because this unit can either aid or complicate all aspects of human resources management.

A library fortunate enough to hire its own human resources administrator may select someone with the qualities outlined by Duda. He identifies differences between line and staff roles for carrying out human resources managerial tasks, arguing that selection criteria for a human resources administrator should be "both as flexible and relevant as possible" [27].

Although staff are the health sciences library's most important resource, Duda states that "it is rare to find a statement of an institution's personnel objective or philosophy." He claims that all organizations have human resources objectives, even if they are implicit, and that these objectives serve to guide managers and human resources administrators. Such objectives "should include a description of governance, staff development programs and opportunities, and staff involvement in the decision-making process" [28].

STAFFING PATTERNS AND ORGANIZATIONAL STRUCTURE

Health sciences libraries range in size from the small, one-person library in a community hospital or research center to libraries with sixty or seventy staff serving the information needs of multiple health disciplines in large academic health centers and hospitals. Among academic health sciences libraries, some share certain functions, such as acquisitions or cataloging, with the general academic libraries on their campuses, while others do not. With such diversity, no single recommendation for optimum staffing is possible.

What is clear is that the library staff must be equipped to function as "knowledge workers" in their own environment. They must be able to assess the information needs of users and respond with appropriate products and services. In any type of health sciences library, meeting this goal will determine the optimum number of staff, their knowledge and abilities, and their responsibilities. This is the essence of human resources planning. In today's climate of continuous change, external factors affect human resources planning. Examples include the impact of information technology on both the nature of work performed and users' expectations, the labor market and economy, affirmative action, and the impact of a civil service system or labor union in the organization.

Standards and guidelines exist for staffing various types of health sciences libraries. These documents call for staffing levels appropriate to meet stated needs. For example, the MLA *Standards for Hospital Libraries* state that

> the library and information services are managed by a qualified medical librarian. Additional medical librarians and support staff may be needed to provide quality services as determined by a needs assessment.

They go on to add that if the medical librarian is serving as a consultant, rather than as a permanent staff member, then the hospital should assign the responsibility of performing routine library operations to another hospital employee [29].

The Association of Academic Health Sciences Library Directors document *Challenge to Action: Planning and Evaluation Guidelines for Academic Health Sciences Libraries* calls for the library to "broaden the ability of library personnel to meet changing needs and improve expertise through recruitment, training and continuing education" [30]. Similar guidelines exist for dental and chiropractic libraries [31-32]. These statements clarify why it is important for a library to have a personnel plan, since each of them places the responsibility on library administrators to set the appropriate level of staffing necessary to meet their users' and institutions' needs.

White points out that the smaller the library, the greater the flexibility needed in any position [33]. He also notes that larger libraries are beginning to use more flexibility in describing duties because distinctions in duties are becoming increasingly blurred. For instance, collection development may be a function assigned to one individual or may be part of the responsibility of several people. Academic reference librarians sometimes serve as liaisons to various health disciplines or constituencies. Their duties may include selecting materials in their liaison areas. Teaching can be the primary function of one or more library staff or shared among staff with various other functional roles. Computer systems support has become so central to all library activities that most libraries now employ staff dedicated to supporting this function. At the same time, a basic level of computing competence is expected from all staff. New staff roles have recently emerged in areas such as the following:

- Consultant librarians perform specialized information services for an individual user or group of users, including delivering repackaged and synthesized information as envisioned in the Matheson Report [34].
- Web managers develop and manage library Web sites and databases and create portals to various information resources and services.
- Librarians use new technologies to develop and deliver instruction to learners through a variety of mechanisms, including distance education.
- Fund-raising experts undertake campaigns to increase libraries' levels of private funding.
- Research and evaluation specialists help libraries assess the quality of their services.
- Subject specialists help launch new knowledge management activities.

Libraries also have been able to assign higher levels of responsibility to support staff, often reassigning duties formerly performed by librarians. Professional librarians then focus on planning, specialized services, and evaluation activities. For example, highly qualified and trained support staff now perform most cataloging functions in many libraries and participate in information system planning and maintenance. This role assignment allows librarians to focus on creating new knowledge databases or planning new information systems or services. In some libraries, support staff provide on-site assistance to users of library information systems, while reference librarians are engaged in information consultation services and teaching. Although the ratio of one-third professional staff to two-thirds support staff still serves as a general standard [35], this ratio varies widely among libraries as continuing changes in professional and support staff roles affect it.

Despite the changes in professional and support staff roles, most libraries still reserve the title of librarian for those who perform tasks that require graduate-level professional training, according to the 1976 recommendations of the American Library Association (ALA) *Library Education and Personnel Utilization* policy [36]. Greer, Agada, and Grover call for a new title, "information manager," to be applied to individuals professionally trained to provide value-added information services. They suggest applying the title "librarian" to trained individuals who perform highly technical support tasks but lack a graduate library degree [37].

Libraries in or near academic institutions typically rely heavily on part-time student workers as an inexpensive part of their workforce. Students can often be recruited who have the cognitive and technical abilities to perform both primary and support roles in most functional areas of the library. However, they may also require considerable on-the-job training, and their commitment is understandably to their academic goals. In general, they do not prove to be as reliable as permanent staff. A library choosing to rely heavily on student workers should consider incentives for retention, such as frequent small wage increases. It is also important to give student workers regular feedback and encourage them to achieve their maximum job performance, just as with any employee.

WORKING IN TEAMS

Many librarians find that, as the nature of their work changes, their library organizational structures change as well. Hierarchical structures give way to matrix- and team-based organizations. The team is a group of people who pool their skills, talents and knowledge to achieve a common purpose. Team characteristics can vary in terms of their duration, permanence, membership, work approaches, and goals. In this respect, library task forces, departments, and committees, as well as other ad hoc groups, constitute teams.

According to one source, teams can be categorized as functional, cross-functional, multifunctional, and networks [38]. A *functional* team in the library could consist of reference or education librarians, whose members have the same basic job and the same skills and who support one another and work closely together. A *cross-functional* team's members have different functions and skills but serve the same client and understand the whole process. This might describe members of a library department, a task force to design a new information system, or a committee to plan a new library building.

In a *multifunctional* team, each member possesses all the skills needed for a process or service; members are cross-trained and have the maximum flexibility to serve clients. Some libraries staff single service points for core user information services (e.g., circulation, basic reference, reserves, and document delivery service) with such multifunctional teams. Finally, a *network* consists of members who work in separate libraries but who share information, collaborate, create joint plans and policies, and may work together in ad hoc teams. Health sciences libraries have many examples of working together in networks, ranging from the National Network of Libraries of Medicine (NN/LM) to local groups that collaborate for joint database licensing, shared training, and other purposes.

Clearly, many library staff members work in teams already. In the future, library staff will very likely work predominantly in teams with other staff, other information professionals, faculty, and library clientele. Why are teams so important in today's health sciences library? Library work has become more complex, requiring expertise in multiple areas. Teams provide opportunities for increased collaboration among experts from various functional areas of the library and, in some cases, will include expertise from outside the library as well. Most library service decisions affect multiple functions within the organization and benefit from broad staff involvement. With the blurring of roles among various types and levels of staff, an increased emphasis is placed on broad staff participation in decision making. These changes add to the complexity of the role of each and every library staff member, but they also provide opportunities for personal growth and leadership development.

Because teams represent a different way of working together, it is important for a library administrator to create and support teams that work effectively and produce desired results. Determining team members may be done in various ways. Selection of members may be based on their knowledge and perspective about the problem. Some choices rely on team role criteria, which focus more on an individual's function in a group than on the individual's specific knowledge or expertise [39]. The best approach to selection depends on the specific organization, the type of team, and the result desired.

Supporting effective teams means making a management investment in team building. Regardless of the purpose or type of the team, its members need to develop the necessary skills to solve problems together. Members require skills in communicating, sharing responsibility, managing the agenda, solving problems, building trust, and other areas. These skills cannot be assumed to exist in staff who are more experienced at working in hierarchical settings. Failure to nurture and develop these skills leads to poor performance or the downfall of many teams, even when the team membership is appropriate. The ongoing training and development of individuals holding support positions is just as important to the library's success as it is for the professional librarians.

Effective teamwork rests on changes to the human resources policies and practices that supported hierarchical management structures. For example, new group evaluation processes may be needed that reward team results and teamwork rather than individual behavior. Collaborative evaluation processes have also been used successfully with techniques such as "360-degree evaluation," in which each team member evaluates every other member anonymously, and the results are compiled and shared.

THE LEGAL FRAMEWORK

Laws and regulations governing the employment and treatment of staff have multiplied over the past several decades. They limit the freedom of the library administrator to make some personnel decisions, yet they also guarantee equitable treatment and better working conditions for staff and promote the goal of achieving diversity in the workplace. Library directors should be aware of major employment legislation and how it affects them, but they also should turn for guidance in its application to the human resources administration and legal counsel of their parent organization.

Title VII of the Civil Rights Act of 1964 prohibits sex discrimination in all aspects of employment and also is the basis for prohibiting sexual harassment. It comprises the most significant antidiscrimination legislation to affect health sciences libraries. This law has contributed significantly to improved working conditions for women. It led to the Pregnancy Discrimination in Employment Act of 1978 that forbids using pregnancy as grounds for discrimination in employment. The Civil Rights Act supports nondiscriminatory terms in the employment, insurance, and leave policies of many organizations. However, it does not protect sexual preference. Numerous attempts in federal courts to claim discrimination under Title VII have been unsuccessful, and the Equal Employment Opportunity Commission (EEOC) has upheld this view. The gay rights movement has obtained this protection occasionally in local legislation. Title VII today applies to virtually all nonfederal libraries.

In the federal sector, the key antidiscrimination executive orders are EO 11478 and EO 11246, which take the further step of requiring federal agencies and government contractors to maintain affirmative action plans. The executive orders require a good faith effort to meet the goals. In 1991, a new Civil Rights Act defined more clearly which actions are discriminatory and how to prosecute them. The 1991 act also called for the Glass Ceiling Initiative, a congressional investigation that reported that significant progress had been made to eliminate barriers to the advancement of women, although many barriers still exist.

The EEOC was created to enforce the Civil Rights Act's provisions, and it also considers sexual harassment as a form of sexual discrimination. It publishes guidelines defining sexual harassment and the conditions under which it might occur and calls for employers to develop procedures for handling complaints. Furthermore, the EEOC encourages employers to educate managers and to take other actions demonstrating the organization's commitment to prevention and correction of any form of sexual harassment. A library director would be well advised to be informed about, and visibly supportive of, the parent organization's sexual harassment prevention program.

Many libraries or their parent organization maintain affirmative action or diversity plans as a result of the Civil Rights Act or executive orders mentioned here. Such plans aim to correct past discriminatory hiring practices, to achieve a more diverse workforce in terms of racial and gender balance, to establish equitable recruitment practices, or to meet the mandated requirement of executive orders. When hiring goals are stated in the plan, they typically reflect the availability of minorities in the labor pool.

Librarians consider affirmative action plans a mixed blessing. Both at the professional librarian and support staff levels, females typically constitute a majority of the library's employees. This makeup can help the parent organization meet a larger hiring goal, but it does not achieve a more diverse library workforce. It is especially challenging to hire racial and ethnic minority librarians in some parts of the country because their presence in the labor pool is quite small. In fact, achieving cultural diversity in libraries generally has met with limited success. Some argue that ways must be found beyond those mandated by law to make our libraries more reflective of a culturally diverse society. Glaviano and Lam, among others, suggest that only through conscious efforts to promote our libraries as environments that welcome diversity will we achieve greater success in recruiting and retaining minority librarians [40].

Current thinking places a high value on diversity in a library organization because it injects fresh perspectives and knowledge [41-42]. If this belief proves true, affirmative action as public policy designed to correct prior discriminatory practice may eventually prove to be unnecessary [43]. However, the public debate about the value of affirmative action begun in California and other states appears certain to intensify in the near future [44].

Legislation governing the collective bargaining process is also of interest to health sciences librarians. This includes the 1935 National Labor Relations Act (also known as the Wagner Act), which assured that management would not interfere with the unionization process in the private sector. Public employees were given the same rights via Executive Orders 10988 and 11491. In 1947 the Taft–Hartley Act amended the Wagner Act to impose greater restrictions on collective bargaining. The inclusion of librarians in collective bargaining units has been variable, appearing to reflect their status within their institutions (e.g., whether they have managerial responsibilities and/or faculty status). The Association of College and Research Libraries' Joint Statement on Faculty Status of College and University Librarians provides a guide for inclusion of librarians with faculty in collective bargaining units [45].

The impact of unions on the library workforce may also result from professional and staff associations that act like unions.

Duda provides an extensive discussion of the collective bargaining process in *Personnel Administration in Libraries* [46]. His discussion includes both contract negotiation and administration. He notes that collective bargaining is often thought to be adversarial and have only negative results. Yet it can help some library organizations move toward a more consultative, participatory management approach, build stronger working relationships between management and staff, bring economic benefits, and improve working conditions overall.

These are, indeed, among the primary reasons that unions have appealed to workers. However, unions' impact is on the wane. Union membership overall has declined from a high of 35% of the U.S. workforce in 1953 to 15% in 1994 [47]. More of today's workforce is likely to be temporary, part-time, in small organizations and companies, and in white-collar and service jobs. Workers have new legislative protection in areas formerly covered only by labor agreements, and increased business competition requires flexibility in staffing that conflicts with most labor contracts [48]. Some labor experts predict a resurgence in union popularity due to the highly competitive business environment. It is not clear how these trends will affect the library workforce.

Other legislation with the potential to affect staff in libraries includes the Occupational Safety and Health Act (OSHA) of 1970. Prior to this act, many states created their own legislation to enforce safe workplaces but were often criticized for being ineffectual. OSHA aims to reduce dangerous working conditions and encourage employers to implement improved safety and health programs. According to OSHA, an organization should have a policy stating its commitment to employee safety and to illness and injury prevention, how hazards will be identified and controlled, and how employees will be made aware of and trained to use safety procedures [49]. Rarely does a hospital or academic health center today operate without such a health and safety program and policy. Library administration should be aware of the policies in their parent organization and strive to enact them in staff's best interests. Environmental concerns in libraries stem from increased interest in health disorders caused by prolonged work with computer screens and sensitivity to indoor air pollutants.

More recently, the Immigration Reform and Control Act of 1986 makes it unlawful to hire an illegal alien. Employers must verify each applicant's eligibility for employment and retain this verification in their records. Librarians should familiarize themselves with the requirements for hiring authorized noncitizens. The Fair Credit and Reporting Act of 1970 and the Privacy Act of 1974 place constraints on information about federal employees that can be stored, used, or released by employers. Some states have enacted similar legislation, while others have open records laws that reduce the individual privacy of state employees. Access to personnel information is increasingly sensitive as such data becomes computer based.

The 1991 Americans with Disabilities Act (ADA) also suggests that changes in hiring practices may be needed to avoid discrimination against individuals with disabilities. The law requires any employer with fifteen or more employees to make "reasonable accommodations" to the limitations of persons who are otherwise qualified.

This discussion only touches on the national legislation most directly affecting personnel decisions in libraries. It is important for library administrators in all types of health sciences libraries to be aware of relevant legislation. Usually human resources administrators in the parent organization can provide needed updates as laws and legal interpretations continue to evolve.

JOB ANALYSIS AND EVALUATION

Most library administrators employ job analysis and evaluation techniques to identify how a job may have changed over time and to evaluate its responsibilities in comparison to other jobs in the library or parent organization. In the rapidly changing library environment, this process is essential to ensure that changes in the level and type of duties are accurately reflected in job descriptions, classifications, and compensation levels. Human resources administrators in the parent organization often oversee or carry out this process with support staff positions. In such cases, it is essential for the library administrator to educate human resources staff about the library's operations. Human resources administrators can gain valuable background about the library by reading its annual report or newsletter, visiting the library, and meeting with staff. This approach will help provide the context to assure that the job analysis efforts for library positions reflect both the nature of work being performed and the setting. Furthermore, library administrators will find job analysis techniques useful prior to filling a vacant position and when reorganizing.

Job analysis consists of collecting data on the actual duties performed and the requirements of a specific position. Creth provides a detailed account of various methods of collecting data, including use of a questionnaire, observations, interviews, and inventorying tasks [50]. She emphasizes the importance of communicating to staff about the purpose and process of job analysis to forestall anxiety and fear over the outcome. The grievance process should be explained in advance of beginning the analysis. One important product of the job analysis is an accurate job description. Creth recommends that the job description should include the following essential elements [51]:

- position title;
- brief summary of major duties (one to three phrases);

- list of major duties performed, in order of importance (these should be stated with action verbs, and include an estimate of the percent of time required for each);
- description of the supervisory role of the position, as well as to whom it reports;
- description of the relationship of the position to other positions in the unit or to other related positions;
- description of the major tools, equipment, and other resources used by the employee;
- statement of the skills and experience required to perform the job.

A *job evaluation* reviews the worth of each job in relation to others. It is useful when creating or updating a classification or compensation plan and employs both quantitative and qualitative techniques. The *ranking* technique ranks all jobs in the library against benchmark jobs at the top and bottom of the organization. A rank is based on a review of the whole job (i.e., the job description), and the criteria are usually subjective. *Job grading* takes a somewhat more objective approach, matching jobs against a predetermined set of criteria. A third approach, the *point system,* is the most commonly used form of job evaluation. It is based on job factors that are important to all library jobs, such as knowledge and skills required and decision making. The evaluator sets a scale of values for each factor, and points are then assigned to each factor in each job being evaluated. A fourth approach, *factor comparison,* begins by evaluating benchmark jobs against factors common to all jobs and then measuring other jobs against the resulting scale. Creth discusses each of these techniques in more detail [52]. McCann et al. describe a job grading process used at the Medical College of Georgia Greenblatt Library. A new job classification system for library support staff was created as a result of their analysis, which helped the library provide a promotional ladder for staff, reduce turnover, and better reflect the evolving complexity of library jobs [53].

Job evaluation techniques prove useful for professional librarian positions as well as for support staff positions. Once jobs are compared, salary ranges can be determined. Where an individual places within that range will depend on experience as well as on the job itself.

A one- or two-person health sciences library may not need to carry out job analysis. However, Roberts describes one instance in which work sampling and analysis in a one-person library helped determine whether to hire a professional librarian or support staff into a vacant position [54]. If the library does not do its own job analysis, the parent organization may employ such techniques, and it is important to be aware of them in order to place library staff equitably within the organization. Particular attention should be paid to positions in the information systems areas of hospitals and academic institutions that may include job factors similar to those in libraries. Once a job analysis is done, the results can be updated through regular performance appraisals and reviews of job descriptions.

RECRUITMENT AND RETENTION OF LIBRARY STAFF

Earlier reference has been made to the importance of recruiting health sciences library workers with the skills and attributes needed to function in today's information-intensive environment. Those key characteristics have also been described. MLA's *Platform for Change* calls for the development of strategies "to recruit bright, articulate, creative, and energetic individuals as health information professionals, including those who pursue formal training as librarians and those who pursue degrees in related disciplines" [55]. What recruitment strategies can a library employ to attract and retain staff with these attributes and skills?

The Association of Academic Health Sciences Libraries' board of directors recommends several strategies, including "developing a strategic vision of the library . . . which transcends traditional roles and expectations . . . ; fostering an atmosphere that encourages individuals' initiative, assumption of responsibility and risk-taking; promoting staff collaboration with other academics in the institution; and committing resources to support staff development programs" [56]. These strategies create an environment in the library that attracts the best-qualified information professionals, and they can be applied in any health sciences library setting. Successful recruitment incorporates numerous steps in the hiring process.

In the first and most important step, the library manager analyzes the position to be filled and updates the position description, if necessary. Filling a vacant position serves as a key opportunity to change reporting relationships, refocus job responsibilities, and bring about organizational change. It affords an opportunity to articulate the critical qualities and skills to be sought in the person hired. Library administrators must be sensitive to the changing character of library staffing and recruit individuals with degrees or expertise in related fields to librarianship, such as medical informatics and education, when doing so can enhance the library's service role.

Recruiting to fill a professional librarian position usually begins with the development of a recruitment plan. The recruitment plan should briefly describe the position to be filled and outline the approach for alerting potential candidates to the vacancy. It identifies the newsletters, newspapers, professional journals, telephone joblines, electronic bulletin boards and listservs, placement services at professional meetings, library schools, professional colleagues, and other personal contacts that are potential recipients of the vacancy announcement. In addition, the vacancy should be posted within the library and organization to notify qualified staff of a promotional opportunity. In most cases, a national search will attract the best applicants. When a local or regional search will suffice to attract applicants, the list of sources can be adjusted accordingly.

Before a recruitment plan can be implemented, it should be reviewed by the library's affirmative action or equal employment opportunity (EEO) officer or by the individual serving in that capacity for the institution or organization. Libraries must make concerted efforts to attract minority candidates, beginning with assuring that the job announcement will receive wide dissemination. The EEO officer will review the plan to assure that it meets this and other objectives, such as diversity in the composition of the search committee and evaluating candidates only on the basis of their qualifications for the position.

Although women constitute over three-fourths of the workforce in health sciences libraries, Anderson suggests that libraries' ability to attract the best candidates is negatively influenced by historical prejudices in the promotion and equitable compensation of women [57]. The poor track record of recruitment of racial and ethnic minorities to library schools further constrains their recruitment into the health sciences setting [58]. Today, the individuals who are sought by libraries are also desired in other information-related fields, so that libraries must advertise and compete more aggressively. MLA maintains an employment opportunities list in each issue of the *MLA News*. In addition, the MLA Jobline provides a telephone listing of job openings, which is frequently updated, and MLA Net aims to provide job vacancy announcements via the Internet. Increasingly, employers are turning to electronic means of listing job openings. Listservs such as MEDLIB-L, PACS-L, AAHSL, and others disseminate job notices widely, instantly, and at no charge. Academic health sciences libraries often list job openings in the *Chronicle of Higher Education*, which results in an automatic simultaneous posting to its electronic job listing, the Chronolog.

The most efficient way to screen applicants for a vacancy is to assign the responsibility to an individual, such as the direct supervisor or a human resources administrator. Wherever practical, however, it is preferable to employ a search committee. This approach provides more staff input into the screening process and offers a valuable learning opportunity for the staff. The library administrator may appoint one search committee that oversees the recruitment for any and all searches conducted over a specified time, such as one year. This allows the members to become familiar with standard procedures, develop expertise in interview techniques and evaluation processes, and learn more about the library's operation and management philosophy.

Another, more common approach is to appoint a search committee for each new search. In this case, the members typically represent the functional and complementary departments of the library or the management level of the position. A search requires support from a personnel administrator who is familiar with the requirements and policies of the library and the parent organization. A clear and complete procedures manual, with samples of letters and other documents used, also assists the committee. The manual should emphasize the importance of confidentiality in all deliberations of the search committee and on the part of any other staff involved in screening candidates.

The search committee compares the applications received with the job description and qualifications sought and arrives at a list of those applicants who warrant an interview. The cover letter and résumé are the two key documents. The importance of the cover letter should not be underestimated. An applicant should provide a well-written summary matching his or her qualifications to the position available and also address motivation for seeking the position. The résumé should be well organized, concise, and easy to read. It should document the applicant's employment history, educational background, and professional involvement as well as identify specific skills and abilities.

During the search, references should always be sought for applicants who are under serious consideration. Contacting references helps identify the short list of those who will be interviewed. Some organizations prefer to wait until after interviews to seek references, however. Whatever the sequence, this important source of information should not be omitted. It is preferable to develop a uniform list of questions to ask references, especially if more than one individual will be making calls. If letters are requested, references should be asked to address areas of experience and skills that are related to the position description. Because letters of reference may be subject to local open records legislation, some individuals will decline to make critical observations in writing, and the search committee must take this possibility into account when deciding how best to obtain accurate and complete information about candidates.

Personal interviews play an important part in the selection process. They allow both the applicant and the library to assess whether there is a good match. For this reason, it is preferable for the applicant to meet as many of the library staff as is reasonable. This also helps convince the candidate that choosing the best person for the vacant position is important to the entire staff, not just to the immediate coworkers. In larger libraries, this process obviously cannot be accomplished through individual interviews with each staff member, while in smaller libraries this approach may be best. Some options for larger settings include a brief presentation by the candidate to all interested staff, followed by an open interview session; group interviews scheduled with selected staff from the department which has the opening; group interviews with selected staff from a cross-section of library functional areas; or invitations to staff to join in meals with the applicant. These approaches, together with individual interviews with the position's supervisor, the director, and perhaps with coworkers in other parts of the organization, produce successful results.

Important steps to preparing for a successful interview include the following:

- Sending candidates an interview schedule and background information about the library, such as the latest annual report, prior to the interview
- Distributing the interview schedule and candidate's résumé or curriculum vitae in advance to staff who will be participating in the selection
- Clarifying the interview responsibilities of each individual and group who will be involved in the interview. This may include preparing in advance specific questions to be asked. It also should include coaching to prevent asking any questions that do not pertain specifically to job responsibilities and the candidate's qualifications.
- Providing the candidate with a brief library tour prior to the actual interview, if time permits

Following the interview, reactions should be sought in writing from all staff who had an opportunity to hear or meet with the candidate. Again, confidentiality is important. According to Wilkinson, the "interviewers should be looking for the one negative factor among many excellent ones, because the one may be all-important" [59]. While success on the job is attributable to many factors, failure may be the result of only one.

The procedures for making an offer of employment vary from one organization to another. Usually the library director or human resources officer calls the preferred candidate to make an informal offer and to discuss salary, starting date, rank (if applicable), and other employment details. In most cases a formal written offer follows, stating terms of employment to which the successful candidate should agree in writing. Final approval from the organization's EEO office may also be obtained. Some institutions require that their chief executives or board of trustees approve offers of faculty-level positions before they become official. In other cases, professional staff unions may require additional steps for approval of an appointment.

Candidates deserve timely information about how the search is proceeding or when it has concluded. Such communication leaves strong impressions of how employees are likely to be treated. Unsuccessful applicants should be notified personally of the outcome of a search. A telephone call is the best way to do this, at least for those candidates who have been interviewed. Others should receive personal letters thanking them for their interest in the library and informing them that the position has been filled.

Recruiting and hiring the best possible staff represents an essential role of the library administrator. Having made the substantial investment in recruitment, no one wants to think about staff turnover and the continuing cycle of recruitment that this implies. Certainly the wise administrator will recognize that retention is as important a human resources role as recruitment. The best way to discover a problem or a potential problem that may be leading to staff turnover is to conduct exit interviews with departing staff. The exit interview provides the employee with a confidential opportunity to disclose his or her reasons for leaving. Some organizations require that a written exit interview report be filed. Even in these cases, a personal exit interview is desirable, because it often results in more forthright and detailed information. Ideally, the supervisor, human resources officer, or the library director should conduct the exit interview. If turnover rates seem unusually high, it may be helpful to track reasons for resignations, to identify trends. Whether the reasons relate to working conditions or personal circumstances, the information gives useful feedback to the library administrator.

Retention of staff will depend on whether the library meets the staff member's expectations, and vice versa. *Challenge to Action* calls for the library to "enhance recruitment and retention of high quality staff by monitoring institutional personnel policies, salaries and benefits to insure that library staff is treated fairly" [60]. However, in even the best libraries, staff turnover can be expected and even welcomed as an opportunity for personal growth, infusion of new perspectives, and reexamination of the library's needs. Some of those expectations, having to do with professional growth, compensation and benefits, evaluating performance, and overall quality of work life, will be discussed briefly in the next section of this chapter.

STAFF TRAINING AND DEVELOPMENT

The library broadens the ability of library personnel to meet changing needs and improves expertise through recruitment, training and continuing education. [61]

Employers should place a high priority on staff development . . . and should provide institution-based training within the context of the broader educational experience [62].

Both MLA and AAHSL, through these statements, emphasize the library's responsibility to ensure that its staff maintains the skills and expertise needed in today's changing information environment. However, the individual and the employer share responsibility for staff development. *Platform for Change* specifies roles for MLA, NLM, and graduate schools of library and information science. These roles recognize the broader responsibilities of creating and sustaining an expert workforce and pursuing collaborative approaches. The majority of the current health sciences library workforce is likely to be in the profession for at least the next fifteen years [63]. If these employees are to maintain the skills required in their changing work environments, continuing education must be of paramount importance.

A library of any size can and should have a systematic staff development program. Doing so ensures that the library staff keeps pace with change and is capable of responding to new directions and new priorities. As Creth points out, "there is not a choice as to whether or not to train and develop staff; there is only a choice of how to approach this responsibility" [64]. Staff will seek the skills they need to perform their work in one way or another. The benefits of a systematic approach include the ability to plan training on the basis of identified needs, monitor the quality of the training and of the resulting work, and build a staff that is uniformly confident, competent, and resourceful.

This is not to diminish the value of unstructured or personally tailored learning pursued by individuals in support of their own learning goals. Health sciences librarians "must assume personal responsibility for aggressively seeking lifelong education and professional development opportunities from a variety of sources," says *Platform for Change* [65]. But *Platform* also calls for a library to maintain a staff development program that "balances institutional needs and the professional growth objectives of the individual." It goes on to call for the library to assist individuals in designing their own professional development program. This program may include specific learning experiences to meet the library's needs, as well as continuing education experiences that address the needs and interests of the individual.

Staff participation in continuing education should be encouraged to the extent that library resources permit. The staff development plan and policy should define guidelines for staff participation in all types of learning activities. In commenting on *Platform for Change*, Creth notes that for a personalized professional development plan to be effective, the individual must welcome continuous learning and the opportunity for change and not view him- or herself as being a victim of the environment. Creth goes on to say that, unfortunately, "too few libraries expend significant resources for professional development and staff training, even though this investment would pay off handsomely in increased staff capacity as measured by competence, confidence, flexibility, and innovation" [66].

The chief components of a staff development program, according to Creth, include orientation, on-the-job training, and development [67]. Continuing education, while often difficult to separate from staff development, is not a formal component of Creth's schema because she defines its purpose as primarily meeting personal interests of the individual, which may or may not benefit the library. However, the library ideally should support continuing education to the extent that resources permit. In such a rapidly changing work environment, employers should value and support an individual's commitment to continued learning, even if it leads to a job change outside the organization.

New Employee Orientation

The staff development program begins with orientation of a new library employee. Orientation should familiarize the employee with the policies and procedures of the library; the overall work environment and the specific job to be performed; and the parent institution, hospital, or other organization of which the health sciences library is a part. Depending on the library, orientation can be carried out by the supervisor, fellow staff members, a personnel administrator, or a combination of these. Because orientation necessarily covers a great deal of information, a checklist is useful to be sure that all relevant information has been covered. The checklist might include a review of position responsibilities, the library's mission and goals, work schedule, introduction to staff and other work colleagues, overview of all library departments and work functions, major library systems, institutional and library policies and procedures, and more.

Many libraries prepare a staff handbook that includes similar information for later referral. It also is helpful to stagger the presentation of this new information over a period of time rather than present it all on the employee's first day. Orientation also serves to socialize a new employee to the culture of the library and the larger organization. An employee must begin to feel as though he or she belongs to, and can contribute to, the library.

Job Training

Job training is the second element of a staff development program. As defined by Creth, job training consists of both formal and informal activities that address the three dimensions of knowledge, skills, and abilities [68]. While it is a continuous process, three distinct opportunities exist for training: for the new employee, for performance improvement, and for learning new or changed library operations or processes. Traditionally a job training plan is prepared and carried out by the employee's supervisor, who is in the best position to observe results. However, as the library work environment changes, so does the environment for training. When a new online system is introduced, for instance, greater benefit derives from centralized training, for both efficiency and the broader perspective that comes from seeing how others use the technology.

Library functional areas are blurring. As cross-functional groups develop, training needs arise that often are best carried out by individuals other than the direct supervisor. For example, some libraries are experimenting with combining multiple public service functions in a single service desk. Staff needing to perform functions ranging from ready reference to technical support to cash handling will require additional training. This creates the challenge of finding ways to maintain the training and performance continuum. Training should bring about a change in performance or behavior. When evaluating training, this changed behavior must be observable.

Employee Development

Development activities are distinguished from skills training by being broader and more conceptual. Examples include stress management, introduction to marketing, or new approaches to document delivery services in an electronic era. Such activities encourage staff to stretch their thinking, examine new attitudes, and envision new approaches. Experts from outside the library often conduct development activities rather than supervisors or personnel administrators. A successful staff development program that includes orientation, job training, and development will address identified needs of the staff and the library. Staff members' days are typically crowded with multiple meetings and the press of an ever-increasing range of duties. Unless staff development activities relate to stated library priorities, staff will be reluctant to participate or will feel frustrated at having to schedule one more activity for which the need is unclear. Consequently, a library should have an explicit staff development plan.

A staff development plan can be created using a basic, commonsense planning approach with steps that

- define the goals and objectives of the staff development program,
- identify development needs,
- determine priorities,
- identify resources, and
- evaluate the activities and the program [69].

The program goals should flow from the library's long-term service priorities. For example, a library priority may aim to provide desktop access to documents for users. A pertinent staff development goal would reflect the need to train and develop staff to provide this service. Likewise, a library priority may describe a conversion from one online library system to another. A staff development goal would then address the need to educate staff to understand the online system's capabilities, train staff to use the new system effectively, and support its use by others. In this way, the staff development plan is continually being revised and updated to reflect the library's needs.

Specific training and development needs can be identified through formal needs assessment of the staff or through other means. Some libraries use the staff performance evaluation process to identify needs. Other ways to determine training needs include a staff survey or recommendations of supervisors based on current library service goals and priorities. Whatever approach is used, the administrator determines the needs most critical to the library and designs activities that respond best to those needs. The activities should encompass the three main areas of orientation, training, and development. Resources used in staff training and development vary widely. The selection depends on many factors, including what is available within the library or parent organization, what funds are available to purchase or rent materials or bring in an outside expert, and factors such as timing, size of the group, and content.

Since library staff are likely to conduct much of the training activities, the effective trainer requires knowledge of the content as well as specific training skills. The staff development plan may use a "train the trainers" approach to distribute the workload and expand the pool of trainers. Within the Association of College and Research Libraries (ACRL), a Personnel Administrators and Staff Development Officers Group maintains an information exchange for training materials and approaches. Similarly, the Association of Research Libraries' (ARL) Office of Management Studies makes available excellent training materials and programs. It helps when library managers tap groups such as these or consult with personnel administrators within the parent organization. Increasingly, sources of training exist within the parent organization, especially as libraries build relationships with other information service providers such as medical informatics and academic computing. As *Platform for Change* notes, one employer responsibility is "discovering, advancing, and tending the learning relationships within and outside the organization" [70].

Whatever training approach is used, a strong staff development plan evaluates results. Each training or development activity should be assessed, for both quality of the teaching/learning process and for its impact. When a staff member attends a training activity outside the library, an evaluative report should be submitted afterward. This feedback facilitates evaluation of the plan itself, as well as of the specific activities. Evaluation of the overall plan should occur periodically to ensure that it addresses the staff's critical learning needs and in the best ways possible.

The creation of a staff development plan and program may seem excessive in a small library with only a few staff. In this context some of the overall objectives may be accomplished informally, through daily contact. In a small health sciences library with less differentiation of functions among staff, each staff member will need to be familiar with multiple functions in greater detail than would be the case in a larger library. In libraries of any size, librarians can increasingly be found interacting with users at the work site, outside the library. These staff are advocates for the library in all of its roles, and must be well informed about them. Staff training and development are important for every health sciences library, but each library should develop an approach customized to its setting.

COMPENSATION AND BENEFITS

MLA has been committed to asserting the professional authority of medical librarians as expert health information professionals. Jacqueline Bastille, 1990-91 MLA president, called attention to the low salaries of medical librarians as one factor that impedes recognition of the value of our profession by society [71]. She suggested how librarians can claim jurisdiction over information management activities in their own institutions, reminding us to continually seek fair and adequate compensation because "salary is an indicator of professional worth and status and, therefore, affects every aspect of our profession and job performance" [72].

MLA's *Platform for Change* also calls for the association to "set the standards for professional competency and compensation" at levels enabling recruitment of individuals who will succeed in the changing technological environment [73]. Working with its Status and Economic Interests of Health Sciences Library Personnel Committee, MLA periodically monitors and reports on salary trends in medical librarianship [74]. The ALA, ARL, AAHSL, and other library associations also report salary trends and support higher salaries, pay equity, and other compensation issues of importance to librarians. A 1992 National Survey of Hospital and Medical School Salaries revealed that the average librarian's salary was lower than the average salary reported for all but two medical professions requiring a master's degree and also lower than the average salary reported for four medical professions requiring only a bachelor's degree. Of the professions surveyed, librarianship was the only one not requiring any qualifications beyond the graduate degree (i.e., licensure or certification) [75].

MLA's 1995 salary survey reports an 8.2% increase in the mean annual salary since the 1992 survey. This report notes a mean salary in 1995 of $40,742 for all respondents, with the mean slightly higher for librarians in academic medical centers compared to those in hospitals. The average entry-level salary for all health sciences librarians was $26,658 [76]. Salary surveys conducted by professional library associations help determine appropriate pay levels according to market factors. State or local salary surveys for support staff may also be available.

Fair and equitable compensation has been, and continues to be, an important issue for the medical library profession as it strives to delineate its critical role in health information management. Compensation is a major factor in attracting and retaining the best qualified workers. Duda states that a compensation program supports recruitment, retention, and pay equity;

rewards good performance; controls costs; complies with legal requirements; and furthers administrative efficiency [77]. Most libraries base compensation on a job classification scheme, as discussed earlier. Such schemes
determine the base level of pay for a given job in comparison to others. The
degree of autonomy given to a library director to establish a classification
and compensation plan varies widely among organizations. Those working
with collective bargaining agreements or in public institutions face external
requirements and constraints.

A library director who establishes or changes a compensation program
should consider what is required to attract and retain the quality of employees
needed. This includes consideration of market factors, union influences, government regulations, budget constraints, and the total compensation package
(base pay, benefits, and merit or performance pay). A compensation plan
should define base pay levels and special pay circumstances, such as differen-
tial pay for evening and weekend work. The plan should outline how pay increases occur, whether through a graded pay system or other means (e.g., promotion or merit). When pay increases are based on merit, it is important to state
performance standards on which merit increases are based and to be consistent and fair in their application. The compensation plan indicates whether
there is a separate pay structure for professional librarians, support staff, and
temporary workers such as students and how these interrelate. The plan describes every job at its appropriate level. Since libraries are part of larger organizations, a compensation expert in the human resources department usually offers guidance in developing an effective compensation plan.

Federal legislation affects compensation for library workers in three key
areas: wage and hour legislation, income protection, and antidiscrimination
legislation. The Fair Labor Standards Act of 1938, with amendments, sets
minimum hourly wage rates and the number of hours an employee may
work without being paid for overtime work. The exclusion of professional
and administrative staff from the provisions of this act means that it does not
apply to librarians, but it does apply to support staff. Income protection legislation includes the Social Security Act and Unemployment Compensation.
As previously mentioned, Title VII of the Civil Rights Act of 1964 prohibits
discriminatory hiring and promotion practices. The Equal Pay Act of 1963
guarantees equal pay for equal work for men and women. Since its enact-
ment, it has not been as successful in achieving pay equity for professional
and management workers as it has been for factory workers. Some states
have instituted their own pay equity studies based on the value or worth of
jobs. ALA and other associations support such studies as a way to eliminate
sex bias in the classification and compensation of library jobs, which are held
principally by females. In several states, such studies have resulted in substantial pay increases for librarians. To date, however, no universally accepted method prevails for determining comparable worth.

Fringe benefits account for an increasing proportion of a total compensation package. The cost of benefits such as health insurance has increased significantly, and workers have sought expanded coverage for other benefits as well. In addition, federal law requires Social Security participation, unemployment insurance, and workmen's compensation. Benefits packages also often include supplemental retirement plans; health, disability, and life insurance; and employee services, such as child care, subsidized housing, and reimbursement for incurred expenses such as travel. Library directors should identify employee benefits they can offer that may not be part of their parent organization's standard benefits package, including support for professional development (e.g., tuition reimbursement or conference registration and travel costs) and financial support for the incidental costs of research projects. Other benefits may not involve additional funding—for example, release time for conference attendance and research activities. Benefits have become an important component to successful recruitment and retention of the best staff.

EVALUATING STAFF PERFORMANCE

Most librarians agree on the value of evaluating staff performance. Well-trained, productive staff are the library's most important resource. A performance evaluation process provides the means for supervisors to offer formal, structured feedback on their employees' performance in support of achieving the libraries' goals. The process can help administrators to

- assess whether staff are being used appropriately;
- recognize special staff skills and praise accomplishments;
- document performance problems and create plans for correcting them;
- formulate upcoming work objectives and describe how individuals will contribute to meeting them;
- identify new training and development needs;
- provide information to support reward and recognition of staff through salary increases, promotions, and other means; and
- help individuals assess their own career development goals.

In short, performance evaluation plays a key role in helping libraries make the best use of the knowledge, skills, and abilities of their staff. While these purposes may be generally recognized as valuable to the library and to the individual worker, there is abundant criticism of how performance evaluation processes are carried out. There are many different approaches to performance evaluation, each with its advocates. And whatever the approach, evaluation can be a difficult process both for supervisors and workers.

Reneker and Steel summarize three reasons for the failure of performance evaluation processes:

- the supervisor lacks objective information on which to evaluate;
- the supervisor has not determined the basis for the evaluation in advance;
- the supervisor is poorly prepared and/or trained to conduct an evaluation [78].

In fact, many librarians become supervisors before they receive training in planning and evaluating job performances; thus, discomfort occurs for both the new supervisor and for the employee being evaluated. Libraries may employ different performance evaluation processes for professional staff and for support staff, often due to the requirement of the parent organization. However, avoiding these common problems can help assure that employees and supervisors benefit from the process.

As rapid change in library roles and functions continues to affect the nature of work performed by staff at all levels, it is critical that staff participate in setting library-wide goals and shaping the specific roles of their work unit. Some performance evaluation processes carry this to the worker's level, developing individual work plans with performance objectives and measures linked to unit goals. Involving staff in this process assures that they are in tune with the library's goals and changes occurring in the library. It also encourages their commitment to achieving the library's goals. Performance expectations can be discussed in advance between the employee and his or her supervisor, and training needs identified.

In assessing performance, the employee's behavior on the job is evaluated in terms of the outcomes or results that behavior produces or influences. It can be difficult to distinguish behavior from abilities or personal characteristics. Behavior is observable, measurable, and related to a desirable job outcome. An example of an observable, measurable behavior is using appropriate online library systems (e.g., DOCLINE and OCLC) to respond accurately to document delivery requests within twenty-four hours of their receipt. Documentable elements of the behavior that can be evaluated include selection of the best system, the location of information needed to respond to the request, and the accuracy and timeliness of the response. The more advance communication between the supervisor and employee about performance expectations, the more accurate and reliable the evaluation process.

Some of the techniques commonly used for performance evaluation in libraries include open-ended essays, behavioral ratings on a scale that differentiates between poor and superior performance, and quantitative and qualitative output measures (e.g., management by objectives). Detailed descriptions of each of these techniques can be found in standard personnel administration texts, some of which are listed in the references at the end of this chapter. Any of the techniques can be applied, periodically updated to reflect current standards, and used alone or in combination with other techniques. In addition, some libraries find that standard proficiency tests, such as those administered by career assessment centers, serve as useful supplements to other techniques for assessing promotion and career development potential.

When any of these techniques is used for personnel decisions, they become subject to the antidiscrimination provisions of Title VII of the 1964 Civil Rights Act and subsequent related court actions. Hodge notes key criteria to consider in developing an evaluation system that will be fair to all employees and useful to management:

- The system is based on job analysis and the enumeration of critical elements in job descriptions and annual performance goals.
- Employees are involved in setting criteria.
- Performance standards are set, for both critical job elements and other important job aspects.
- There is minimal evaluation of personal traits, which can introduce substantial subjectivity by the evaluator.
- Precise, unambiguous language is used in all evaluation forms.
- Where various measures are used, the relative weight of each is clearly determined.
- All managers/supervisors complete training programs on conducting effective performance appraisals [79].

Should performance standards be set for professional librarians as well as for library support staff? This question has been debated by many. Some state that, while professional performance standards are difficult to express, intrinsic standards exist in the minds of librarians in judging their own performance and that of their peers. Some libraries have succeeded in articulating these standards. Federal libraries have done so to be in compliance with requirements of the 1978 Civil Service Reform Act.

Evaluation Options

Traditionally, the employee's direct supervisor has conducted a performance evaluation on the assumption that the supervisor best knows what is expected of the employee and how well those expectations have been met. Today, library staff members increasingly work in teams to develop and provide services. Developing online library systems, providing campus or network document delivery services, sharing collection development responsibilities, or offering clinical information management or education services exemplify efforts that typically involve staff from various parts of the library. Other team members may be faculty or staff from elsewhere in the school, hospital, or larger organization. Whether these are permanent or temporary group structures, they raise questions about performance evaluation. What if the supervisor is not in a position to observe an employee's work in another group? Will an individual's evaluation be based on overall group performance or on the individual's role in the group? The employee and the supervisor should resolve these questions prior to involvement in the group, so that expectations are clear.

Several approaches to team evaluation work successfully. In *360-degree evaluation,* each person anonymously evaluates every other person, and the results are compiled into a confidential report for each team member. In another approach, each team member evaluates two other members, one chosen by the employee and one picked by the rest of the team. The team evaluation seeks to improve team performance. As with any job, evaluation should be based on measurable results and the team's objectives. This is especially important to keep in mind in team evaluation because members' roles may change in the course of the team's work. Cherrington elaborates on more aspects of team evaluation [80].

Peer review works well in evaluating the performance of teams. It has been used traditionally in academic libraries to evaluate librarians who have either faculty or professional status [81]. In both applications, members of a group evaluate the behavior and accomplishments of the other members of the group on the assumption that critical aspects of one individual's work are best observed and judged by the others. It may incorporate information submitted by individuals outside the group and usually is only one part of a larger evaluation process.

Peer review has many recognized inadequacies. Frequent criticisms include concern that it will be a popularity contest, peers mistrust one another, peers are unable to be objective reviewers, and negative reviews will result in reprisals to the reviewers. Reneker and Steel state that a committee can judge but not improve performance [82]. They assert that the most effective evaluation for improving performance is frequent, ongoing feedback from the supervisor. However, library staff working together in teams also depend on good, ongoing communication and coordination of efforts toward reaching shared goals. One challenge to the effectiveness of teams is developing their ability to monitor and guide the performance of each member. As the popularity of group and team efforts increases, staff need to develop team effectiveness skills. These include the ability to evaluate both group and individual performance.

In some libraries, external reviews by supervisors and/or peers are supplemented by self-ratings. Here, too, opinion differs as to their value. Self-ratings are not objective, but Reneker notes that by focusing on the evaluation criteria in judging his or her own performance, an employee's performance may improve. The evaluation interview can be an active discussion, one of joint problem solving [83].

Effective performance evaluation depends on having an atmosphere of trust and open communication in the library. This ensures that employees know on what basis they are being evaluated and how. These criteria must be communicated explicitly and in advance, and they should form the basis of all written material and the discussion during the evaluation dialogue. Evaluation interviews should be scheduled in advance. Both supervisor and employee should have ample time to review the documentation and to plan the points they wish to make. Cherrington notes the popular "sandwich" approach, which places any criticism in between praise at the beginning and end of the interview, thereby creating an overall positive experience to the interview [84], but not all employees deal well with such mixed messages. Effective interviews are private, confidential, unhurried, and take a problem-solving approach, rather than a judgmental approach. One outcome should be a mutual commitment to meeting personal performance goals during the upcoming review period, with both the employee and supervisor having a stated role in the achievement of those goals. All employees should be trained to participate actively in the performance evaluation process. They should understand its importance to achieving the library's goals and to optimizing their own performance.

Handling Performance Problems

Even the best-prepared library administrators encounter difficult performance problems. For this reason library administrators should be aware of their organization's employee grievance and disciplinary policies and procedures and the support available to make use of them. If a union is present, the labor agreement often spells out the processes. Grievance procedures provide a way to fairly hear and assess the concerns of employees, while disciplinary procedures offer management a means to deal with problem employees. Discipline strives to correct unacceptable employee behavior or, if necessary, to terminate the employee. Both processes serve to balance the needs of management and employees.

Grievance procedures usually involve at least three steps:

1. The employee submits a complaint to the supervisor for discussion.
2. If the grievance is unresolved, an appeal goes to the next higher level in the unit, usually in writing.
3. If still unresolved, the grievance may go to binding arbitration by a mutually acceptable outside party.

Usually a time limit exists for addressing complaints at each level. An organization should seek to resolve as many grievances as possible at the first level [85].

Disciplinary actions can be constructive rather than punitive. The supervisor calmly explains the nature of the employee error and why it is unacceptable. The most common grounds for disciplinary action include breaking rules, insubordination, poor performance, illegal acts, or personal problems. Progressive discipline begins with verbal warnings that proceed, if unresolved, to written reprimands, suspension, and finally discharge. Grievance and disciplinary processes offer a prescribed course of action that should be followed consistently in all applicable cases, and they balance the needs of management and employees.

STRESS AND THE QUALITY OF WORK LIFE

The quality of work life (QWL) concerns many managers. In business, QWL proponents expect that improving the work environment will improve employee productivity and thus revenues. QWL programs may include some or all of these goals: increasing employee participation in decision making, sharing financial incentives, increasing job security, or supporting professional growth and development [86]. For libraries, QWL advocates believe that improving employee satisfaction will improve productivity and therefore the quality of library services. In the highly demanding environment in which health sciences libraries face daily challenges of adapting services to meet constant changes in health care and technology, management strives to maintain a satisfied workforce. Administrators provide staff with a clear involvement in library decision making and show a commitment to staff training and professional development. Both of these factors help employees feel anchored in a rapidly changing environment.

Another consideration gaining importance is alternative work patterns and schedules. For instance, teleworking from off-site is becoming a mainstream way of working. Staff are able to serve on teams or "knowledge communities" that stay in touch electronically and do not meet physically. This changes human resources strategies significantly because it can improve the quality of work life for employees who desire flexibility in work schedules and physical location [87].

Another QWL issue for libraries is stress. Beehr and Fenlason define *stress* as "uncertainty times importance times duration" [88]. These terms apply either to a job or the person in the job. Librarians, as members of a service profession, share vulnerability to additional job-related stress and burnout. They can suffer from exhaustion caused by continuous, emotionally demanding involvement with their public. Many authors call attention to this potential problem for librarians. In her 1991 monograph *Stress and Burnout in Library Service*, Caputo provides a comprehensive account of conditions leading to stress among librarians and offers suggestions for handling it [89].

She noted that surveys conducted in the 1980s confirmed that librarians were experiencing burnout to a considerable degree. The surveyors found that librarians experience many of the stressors common to members of other professions: anxiety over rapid technological changes, budget cuts, heavy workloads, poor management, obnoxious patrons, shifting priorities, discrimination, lack of involvement in decision making, and working nights and weekends [90]. In addition, stressors specific to health sciences librarianship can include the general atmosphere of urgency in a health care setting requiring rapid delivery of information and documents and a high level of accountability for providing current and accurate information. All library employees feel stress caused by confusion (and excitement) over their roles and job expectations as the nature of library work changes dramatically. Finally, it seems librarians work harder and are busier than ever before!

What can be done to cope with these stressors? Caputo describes symptoms and stages of burnout and suggests several self-tests that can help an individual identify his or her vulnerability to burnout on the basis of both personal habits and work environment. She offers a basic plan:

- recognize that stress is a problem,
- take responsibility for dealing with it,
- identify a strategy or strategies that will work for you (by eliminating, reducing, or accepting the sources of stress), and
- develop coping skills.

Coping skills will vary with the individual and the situation, ranging from relaxation techniques to changing jobs. Common suggestions for employees include better time management, improved diet/nutrition, increased physical activity, meditation, and yoga [91].

Caputo also offers tips for library management. Supervisors need to be sensitive to the potential impact of stress on the library workforce. Setting realistic goals, giving frequent feedback, providing needed job training and professional development, showing flexibility in adopting changes to work, and creating an organizational climate that is supportive of employee participation help a manager to minimize the effects of stress.

One common source of stress among library staff today is the need to balance the broader demands of personal life with those of a career. It is the norm, rather than the exception, for a librarian to have commitments to a working partner, children, aging parents, and/or the community. This lifestyle means daily juggling to meet the demands of a stressful job as well as those of a family. The demands of a two-career relationship may lead to decisions to alternate job moves or to engage in long-distance parenting, which creates added stress. Whatever approach is taken, experts agree that setting personal goals and priorities helps achieve balance as much as setting job-related goals and priorities.

Some working partners decide to postpone starting a family, for example. Others are able to hire domestic help, work part-time, work a flexible schedule, or work from home. As previously mentioned, teleworking makes many of these options more feasible than they were in the past. Also, the increasingly popular cafeteria-style benefits programs may offer additional options for meeting dependent care needs and others. Organizing household responsibilities and delegating them among family members also helps relieve the tensions inherent in the "superparent" syndrome. Parents who are flexible and willing to compromise devise creative solutions to time management and keep their personal, family, and professional goals in balance [92-93].

FUTURE ISSUES

Significant pressures will continue to affect the nature of library work and the staff who perform it. The health care industry is driven to demonstrate quality health outcomes at affordable cost in an increasingly competitive marketplace. Employers need to obtain and reward contributions of employees from all parts of the organization to improve the quality or reduce the costs of services or products. This emphasis gives rise to less hierarchical organizational structures and to employee empowerment. The workforce faces continued concern for job security, adequate compensation, equitable hiring practices as affirmative action laws are challenged, and the needs of an aging population. These factors all contribute to significant changes in how work is accomplished.

Such pressures affect health sciences library employees as well. In the future, libraries will operate with staff who possess a high degree of technical skill and, in some cases, advanced knowledge in a health or other discipline. Technology has already routinized some jobs, to the point that they can be carried out from remote locations on behalf of multiple customers. This trend will continue, in particular due to cost-cutting pressures, such as those leading to outsourcing of cataloging. At the same time, technology greatly expands the domain of librarians. Today's library jobs are more technology-intensive and require a more complex level of information analysis, synthesis, and decision making. Library staff must have the ability to apply these skills productively in multifunctional groups and teams.

The greatest challenge for the future will be to create and sustain a workforce that is educated, creative, communicative, energetic, service oriented, and risk-tolerant. Health sciences libraries and information management organizations must attract staff who are both analytical and conceptual, comfortable with ambiguity, and flexible. Such individuals must be committed to continual lifelong learning, for their jobs will change almost daily. They will thrive in an environment in which excitement comes from managing the information and knowledge central to health care delivery, education, and research. Despite the dramatic changes occurring in health care funding, health care delivery systems, health sciences education and research, information management, and the role of the librarian remain as central components. Staff will continue to be the health sciences library's most critical asset.

New health knowledge workers will arise to work alongside the health sciences librarian. There will undoubtedly be competition and some blending of roles with health informaticists, educators, systems developers, systems managers, and others. In this fluid environment, the value of the master's degree in librarianship as a professional minimum requirement will continue to be scrutinized, and the boundaries between professional and support staff will shift yet again. Undergraduate information science degrees are gaining in popularity. As work changes, library administrators will need to be attentive to all of the areas touched upon in this chapter to attract and retain the high caliber staff who will fulfill the library's evolving mission.

REFERENCES

1. Matheson NW, Cooper JAD. Academic information in the academic health sciences center: roles for the library in information management. Washington, DC: Association of American Medical Colleges, 1982:13.

2. Sethi AS, Schuler RS. Human resources management: a strategic choice model. In: Sethi AS, Schuler RS, eds. Human resource management in the health care sector: a guide for administrators and professionals. New York: Quorum Books, 1989:1-14.

3. Welborn RB. The role of organizational development in the strategic human resources management model. In: Sethi AS, Schuler RS, eds. Human resource management in the health care sector: a guide for administrators and professionals. New York: Quorum Books, 1989:221-34.

4. Zuboff S. In the age of the smart machine: the future of work and power. Oxford: Heinemann, 1988:243.

5. Braude RM. Impact of information technology on the role of health sciences libraries. Bull Med Libr Assoc 1993 Oct;81(4):408.

6. Matheson, op. cit.

7. Physicians for the twenty-first century: report of the Project Panel on the General Professional Education of the Physician and College Preparation for Medicine. Washington, DC: Association of American Medical Colleges, 1984.

8. The NLM long range plan: report of the Board of Regents. Bethesda, MD: National Institutes of Health, 1987.

9. Medical education in the information age: proceedings of the symposium on medical informatics. Washington, DC: Association of American Medical Colleges, 1986.

10. Platform for change: the educational policy statement of the Medical Library Association. Chicago: Medical Library Association, 1991.

11. The NLM long range plan on the education and training of health sciences librarians. Bethesda, MD: National Institutes of Health, 1995.

12. Lucier RE. Towards a knowledge management environment: a strategic framework. Educom Rev 1992 Nov/Dec;27(6):24-31.

13. Molholt P. Libraries and the new technologies: courting the Cheshire cat. Libr J 1988 Nov 15;113(19):37-41.

14. Medical Library Association. Value of the hospital library. Chicago: Medical Library Association, 1993.

15. Anderson R. Reinventing the medical librarian. Bull Med Libr Assoc 1989 Oct;77(4):323-31.

16. Ibid., 329.

17. Roper FW, Mayfield MK. Surveying knowledge and skills in the health sciences: results and implications. Bull Med Libr Assoc 1993 Oct;81(4):396-407.

18. Platform for change, op. cit., [11-7].

19. Bowden VM, Olivier ER. The first professional position: expectations of academic health sciences library employees. Bull Med Libr Assoc 1995 Apr;83(2):238-9.

20. Roper FW, Mayfield MK, eds. Symposium: platform for change: medical library education in the information age. Bull Med Libr Assoc 1993 Oct;81(4):393-432.

21. University of Washington Health Sciences Libraries online job posting for associate director for education and consultation, February 4, 1999.

22. Jacobson S. Reorganization: premises, processes, and pitfalls. Bull Med Libr Assoc 1994 Oct;82(4):369-74.

23. Platform for change, op. cit., [19-26].

24. The NLM long range plan, op. cit.

25. Johnson FE, ed. Symposium: NLM planning grants for the education and training of health sciences librarians. Bull Med Libr Assoc 1996 Oct;84(4):514-68.

26. Creth SD, Duda F, eds. Personnel administration in libraries. 2nd ed. New York: Neal-Schuman, 1989.

27. Duda F. Management and personnel administration. In: Creth SD, Duda F, eds. Personnel administration in libraries. 2nd ed. New York: Neal-Schuman, 1989:10.

28. Ibid., 5.

29. Medical Library Association. Hospital Libraries Section Standards Committee. Standards for hospital libraries. Chicago: Medical Library Association, 1995.

30. Joint Task Force of the Association of Academic Health Sciences Library Directors and the Medical Library Association. Challenge to action: planning and evaluation guidelines for academic health sciences libraries. Chicago: Medical Library Association, 1987:9.

31. Medical Library Association. Dental Section. Guidelines for libraries serving dental education programs. Chicago: Medical Library Association, 1992.

32. Medical Library Association. Chiropractic Library Section Standards Committee. Standards for chiropractic college libraries. Chicago: Medical Library Association, 1996.

33. White HS. Library personnel management. White Plains, NY: Knowledge Industry, 1985:5.

34. Matheson, op. cit., 35.

35. Creth, op. cit., 42.

36. American Library Association. Library education and personnel utilization: a statement of policy. Chicago: Office of Library Personnel Resources, American Library Association, 1976.

37. Greer RC, Agada J, Grover R. Staffing: a model for libraries and other information agencies. Libr Admin Manage 1994 Winter;3(1):35-41.

38. Miller LM. Whole system architecture beyond reengineering: designing the high performance organization. Atlanta: Miller Howard Consulting Group, 1994:215-9.

39. Leigh A. Effective change: 20 ways to make it happen. London: Institute of Personnel Management, 1988:193.

40. Glaviano C, Lam RE. Academic libraries and affirmative action: approaching cultural diversity in the 1990's. Coll Res Libr 1990 Nov;51(6):513-23.

41. Thomas RR. From affirmative action to affirming diversity. Harvard Bus Rev 1990 Mar-Apr;90(2):107-17.

42. Thomas DA, Ely RJ. Making differences matter: a new paradigm for managing diversity. Harvard Bus Rev 1996 Sep-Oct;96(5):79-90.

43. Terpstra DK. Affirmative action: a focus on the issues. Labor Law J 1995 May;46(5):307-13.

44. Hodgins L. Rethinking affirmative action in the 1990's: tailoring the cure to remedy the disease. Baylor Law Rev 1995 Summer;47(3):815-39.

45. ACRL standards for faculty status for college and university librarians: a draft revision. Coll Res Libr News 1990 May;(5):402-4.

46. Duda F. Labor relations. In: Creth SD, Duda F, eds. Personnel administration in libraries. 2nd ed. New York: Neal-Schuman, 1989:247-303.

47. Cherrington DJ. The management of human resources. 4th ed. Upper Saddle River, NJ: Prentice Hall, 1995:537.

48. Ibid., 538.

49. Ibid., 631.

50. Creth SD. Personnel planning and utilization. In: Creth SD, Duda F, eds. Personnel administration in libraries. 2nd ed. New York: Neal-Schuman, 1989:72.

51. Ibid., 76.

52. Ibid., 80-4.

53. McCann JC, Davis SE, Trainor DJ. Restructuring support staff classification levels for academic health sciences library positions. Bull Med Libr Assoc 1990 Jul;78(3):293-301.

54. Roberts JT. Work sampling in a one person library. Bull Med Libr Assoc 1994 Apr;82(2):216-8.

55. Platform for change, op. cit., [21].

56. Suggestions for implementing Platform for change. AAHSLD News 1994;14(1):5.

57. Newcomer AP, Pisciotta RA. Career progression of academic medical library directors. Bull Med Libr Assoc 1989 Apr;77(2):185-95.

58. Anderson, op. cit., 326.

59. Wilkinson BR. Recruitment and selection. In: Creth SD, Duda F, eds. Personnel administration in libraries. 2nd ed. New York: Neal-Schuman, 1989:113.

60. Joint Task Force, op. cit., 9.

61. Ibid.

62. Platform for change, op. cit., [24-5].

63. Roper FW, Mayfield MK, op. cit., 404.

64. Creth SD. Staff development and continuing education. In: Creth SD, Duda F, eds. Personnel administration in libraries. 2nd ed. New York: Neal-Schuman, 1989:120.

65. Platform for change, op. cit., [19].

66. Creth SD. The health information environment: a view of organizational and professional needs and priorities. Bull Med Libr Assoc 1993 Oct;81(4):417.

67. Creth SD. Staff development, op. cit., 125.

68. Ibid., 126.

69. Ibid., 130.

70. Platform for change, op. cit., [10].

71. Bastille JD. Elevating the authority of the health information professional: inaugural address. Bull Med Libr Assoc 1993 Jan;81(1):117-9.

72. Bastille JD. Salaries and professional authority: new jurisdictions. Bull Med Libr Assoc 1993 Jan;81(1):80-1.

73. Platform for change, op. cit., [22-3].

74. Health sciences librarian compensation: the results of MLA's 1995 salary survey. Chicago: Medical Library Association, 1995.

75. Neely DM. How do our salaries compare? MLA News 1994 Jan;(261):14.

76. Health sciences librarians' salaries increase. MLA News 1995 Nov/Dec; (280):41.

77. Duda F. Compensation management. In: Creth SD, Duda F, eds. Personnel administration in libraries. 2nd ed. New York: Neal-Schuman, 1989:223-4.

78. Reneker M, Steel V. Performance appraisal: purpose and techniques. In: Creth SD, Duda F, eds. Personnel administration in libraries. 2nd ed. New York: Neal-Schuman, 1989:156.

79. Hodge SP. Performance appraisals: developing a sound legal and managerial system. In: Lindsey JA, ed. Performance evaluation: a management basic for librarians. Phoenix: Oryx Press, 1986:59.

80. Cherrington, op. cit., 299-300.

81. Horn J. Peer review for librarians and its application in ARL libraries. In: Lindsey JA, ed. Performance evaluation: a management basic for librarians. Phoenix: Oryx Press, 1986:82.

82. Reneker, op. cit., 193.

83. Ibid., 189.

84. Cherrington, op. cit., 300.

85. Ibid., 584-6.

86. Stamps PL, Duston TE. The role of quality of work life in the strategic human resources management model. In: Sethi AS, Schuler RS, eds. Human resource management in the health care sector: a guide for administrators and professionals. New York: Quorum Books, 1989:177-91.

87. Taylor JA, McIntosh HD. Managing human resources in the information age. In: Towers B, ed. The handbook of human resources management. 2nd ed. Cambridge, MA: Blackwell, 1996:382-3.

88. Beehr TA, Fenlason KJ. The experience and management of work-related stress. In: Ferris GR, Rowland KM, Buckley MR. Human resource management: perspectives and issues. 2nd ed. Boston: Allyn and Bacon, 1990:391.

89. Caputo JS. Stress and burnout in library service. Phoenix: Oryx Press, 1991:60.

90. Ibid., 62.

91. Beehr, op. cit., 391.

92. Laynor B. Librarianship and motherhood: a part time solution. Med Ref Serv Q 1987 Winter;64(4):15-25.

93. Cochran JW. Time management handbook for librarians. New York: Greenwood Press, 1992.

4

Marketing Library Services

Joan S. Ash and Elizabeth H. Wood

The current marketing concept approach places paramount importance on the needs of the patron/client/customer/user. We use these terms interchangeably for the people libraries serve, but the word *user* will appear most frequently in this chapter. The marketing concept contrasts with the older selling concept, the latter focused on the interests of the seller rather than the buyer. The newer concept of total marketing concentrates on serving the user and his or her needs. This change in thinking has come about for a variety of reasons, but chiefly because most successful companies have shown the new approach simply works more effectively.

At its most basic level, successful marketing depends on good word of mouth. On the average, "a satisfied customer tells three people about a good product experience, [but] a dissatisfied customer gripes to eleven people" [1]. Bad news clearly spreads faster than good. The magnitude of the difference is especially important to health science librarians because each time a library has a dissatisfied customer, librarians are not the only ones who lose. In a clinical context, the library can lose a supporter, but the patient, as the ultimate consumer, stands to lose the most. Patients have now become the direct recipient of library services and are therefore even more the ultimate beneficiaries of excellent service.

Marketing and library professionals have much in common. They both work in the communication arena. Marketers are "skilled at understanding, planning, and managing exchanges" [2]. Librarians and marketers share essentially the same purpose. Both professions have been misunderstood, however; their images have been dramatized and exaggerated negatively in the popular media. Marketing professionals have been portrayed as manipulative charlatans while librarians have been characterized as dull "keepers of the books." Both professions are consciously updating their images at the beginning of the twenty-first century. With more marketing expertise, librarians can more emphatically communicate the importance of their professional knowledge and contributions to their institutions and society at large.

Marketing encompasses numerous specialty areas, including promotion, advertising, and research. In the past the differences between marketing specialties were emphasized, yet the specialties share the same customer focus and can be blended together. This combined approach to the customer orientation parallels integrated approaches to health information delivery and, not surprisingly, benefits from modern electronic marketing information systems.

In *Marketing Is Everything* [3], McKenna contends that everyone in an organization has a marketing role to play. Librarians tend to think of those in technical services functions as being out of the public environment, while front-line staff in public view are expected to give excellent service. However, all library staff must adopt a customer orientation when a user requests a book that has been recently received but not yet processed. Just as the research and development staff in large companies benefit from knowledge of the customer's needs and wants, so does the library's research and technical processing staff. McKenna is right: the marketing concept has to permeate all parts of the organization. As Sherman states, "In the last analysis, developing an image of libraries and librarians rests upon certain principles of packaging and performance" [4]. Marketing the library as a resource for the future necessitates a new point of view toward users [5].

GENERAL CONSIDERATIONS

The objectives of this chapter are to help the reader address the following issues and questions, all of which involve marketing:

- *Time and workload:* If the library staff can't get everything done now, why should they want to market services and increase business? Is it a waste of budget, time, and other resources to develop business a library doesn't need or want?
- *Budget:* How can librarians change a tradition of low pricing? What if the budget is too small to subsidize new services and the library can't charge enough to cover costs?
- *Fees for service:* What about the fee/free dichotomy? If users are accustomed to charges for some services but not others, how will they respond to fees for services that are now free?

- *Clientele:* How can the library define the external market and provide outreach? Does the library have a moral obligation to serve everyone?
- *Expectations:* Can expectation management be handled diplomatically when users want more service and think the library should branch into new areas?
- *Type of library:* Should marketing techniques differ for different kinds of libraries? Do hospital librarians have an advantage in that they know their users better? Do academic health sciences librarians have more resources to put into marketing efforts?
- *Organizational structure:* What marketing can be done in a large, integrated organization? What if the library already has a strong philosophy of service, but some of the other institutional units are more concerned with technology or research?

WHAT IS MARKETING?

Kotler, whose texts include several on marketing nonprofit entities, professional services, and health care services, states:

Marketing is the analysis, planning, implementation, and control of carefully formulated programs designed to bring about voluntary exchanges of values with target markets for the purpose of achieving organizational objectives. It relies heavily on designing the organization's offering in terms of the target markets' needs and desires, and on using effective pricing, communications, and distribution to inform, motivate, and service markets [6].

Marketing strategies have traditionally included the "four *P*s" of price, promotion, place, and product. While recent thinking might add others such as power and politics, the basic four remain valid. Wasserman and Ford explain that "development of a complete marketing strategy entails the awareness of the characteristics and needs of potential customers (patrons, clients or users) and blending the organization's products and services, promotional efforts, pricing, and distribution strategies, to maximize the probability of exchange" [7]. Libraries have used these marketing precepts for years. Their efforts will improve, however, by incorporating some of the tools used by marketing professionals.

WHY MARKETING IS IMPORTANT
FOR HEALTH SCIENCES LIBRARIES

Marketing plays a significant role in highlighting the various foci of the health sciences library. Several of those will be discussed next.

Focus on the User

Libraries must adopt an approach that is customer rather than organization centered if they are to compete with other departments for support. Users need to see the library less as a "combination of diverse and distinct benefits that satisfy specific needs" [8]. As marketing moves away from its older selling orientation toward today's user-oriented concept, it also becomes more useful to libraries and other nonprofit organizations. Marketing fits with librarians' values and beliefs in promoting services for achieving the goal of better health care. If "marketing management's task is to influence the level, timing, and character of demand in a way that will help the organization achieve its objectives" [9], then it can even help librarians cope with the problem of "too much business."

Focus on Service

Health sciences librarians must focus on market research and the product life cycle and must reevaluate constantly the products, services, and marketing strategy to function as a learning organization [10]. User surveys have been a traditional market research tool. Unfortunately, most libraries do not conduct them often enough or consider them as continuous feedback tools. However, librarians do have a great deal of data available about which services and products are most used and by whom [11-12]. By taking the time to analyze and study the data, librarians can also make helpful inferences. Libraries could more effectively use data in areas such as collection use, circulation, database searches, and reference questions.

Focus on the Future

Librarians can no longer assume that library products are valuable and that users will seek them out for their intrinsic value. The librarians' belief system has been "firmly rooted in the idea of the essential nature and unquestioned usefulness of their stock in trade—information" [13]. Consequently, they are jolted when research results indicate that physicians consult colleagues and the *Physician's Desk Reference* before the library [14-15]. Marketing positions the library for success in years to come.

Focus on the Patient

The library's information literacy program is underutilized when health care professionals do not think of the library as their first source of clinical information. Libraries may never replace colleagues as the first source, but they can use marketing techniques to persuade users of the library's important role. When studies demonstrate that even the most difficult patient care questions can be answered by the medical literature 42% of the time [16], librarians need to publicize this information. They need to focus on the opportunity that new technology offers to give rapid responses and quality information [17].

> Librarians must keep current with developing technology and even be anticipatory about its future. . . . Librarians must become more proactive and increase outreach activity [18].

Both legal and social forces are enabling patients to examine their own medical records, perform their own literature searches, and demand more open communication from caregivers. Librarians can not only assist patients in these endeavors but also guide them to resources and teach them to use and evaluate information. Patient education and consumer health have become important to libraries in recent years due to the movement to managed care, the advent of the more informed patient, and easy access to information on the Internet. Commercial promotion of the World Wide Web and its availability in public libraries have encouraged every citizen to become better informed about health issues. Librarians are ideally suited to assisting in this effort. The attractiveness of this medium can be a major promotional tool for all types of libraries [19-20].

Focus on Advocacy

If librarians convince stakeholders that the library is indispensable, it can receive the support necessary to curtail budget cutbacks. Stakeholders include people who use the library, who work in it, who help fund it, who sell products and services to it, to whom it sells products or services, or who influence decisions about it. For example, house staff, faculty, students, and staff may make up the library's active user base, but the financial officer, hospital administrator, auxiliary officer, state governor, or senator may influence funding decisions just as much or more. Rummel and Pence believe that "although we librarians have few natural enemies, neither do we have many natural supporters" [21]. Librarians need to find and create potential supporters; they need to promote themselves, their skills, and their services. Leerburger describes how public libraries have found marketing to be extremely effective: "In all cases in which the public stood behind the library and rejected cuts in funding, there was evidence of a successful marketing effort on behalf of the library" [22].

Focus on Proactive Planning

A marketing plan constitutes an essential part of a complete strategic planning process. In reality, many libraries do not have a written strategic plan [23].

If the parent institution lacks a written plan, it may seem futile to develop one for the library because the plan cannot be tied into broad institutional goals. Fortunately, the National Library of Medicine (NLM) has promoted the development of strategic plans through its Integrated Advanced Information Management Systems (IAIMS) funding, and this program has influenced many organizations beyond those receiving IAIMS funding. Hospital librarians who have promoted their libraries successfully have usually had well-defined plans. They know, for example, the percentage of their target market comprised by nurses or physicians. A marketing plan can exist without an overarching strategic plan, but it cannot be as effective because the context and goals will not be clearly defined.

Focus on Competency

Marketing educates both users and nonusers [24]. It represents one of the library's main communication vehicles. Rapid technological change causes frequent changes in services, makes it difficult for library staff to keep up with change, and introduces even more problems for users who rarely take advantage of library services [25-26]. Through marketing the health sciences librarian both convinces users of the library's value and provides them with current knowledge and information skills.

FUNDAMENTALS OF A MARKETING PLAN

The following discussion outlines a marketing plan, which can be developed at a departmental or library-wide level [27]. The outline and the final result will derive largely from the planning process. Involving more and different types of people produces better results. Staff at all levels and, if possible, other stakeholders as well should be included. The final product will contain both a situation analysis and a multifaceted plan. In the situation analysis, one documents the library's current circumstances. The development of this picture of the present state of affairs can be enlightening and foster consensus building.

The situation analysis commonly describes six elements:

1. *Unit definition:* Planners begin by defining what services the library includes and identify service boundaries. If boundaries are fuzzy, acknowledging this very fact is the first step toward change.
2. *List of products/services the library provides and current clients:* Developing this section of the analysis presents more difficulty than one might expect. Traditionally, products are defined as tangible objects and services as intangibles, but even in the commercial sector a blend-

ing of the two has become more common. For example, verbal assistance and written documentation may serve the same purpose but be defined variously as a service or a product depending on the context and intent of the library.

3. *Outline of the unit's strengths and weaknesses:* This includes skills of staff, major equipment, physical surroundings, or availability of resources.

4. *Analysis of competitive position:* This includes a description of competitors, pricing differences, and other departments that compete for funds [28]. One useful approach includes a table of important competitive qualities with ratings of the home unit and competitors. For example, the library's document delivery turnaround time may be rated on a scale of 1 to 5 and compared with that of a commercial service.

5. *List of environmental trends:* This list includes everything from the budget crisis on campus to national health care reform. It also should include information on predicted demand for library products and services.

6. *List of issues/problems to be addressed by plan:* After completing elements one to five, the planners may elect to create targets. The issues may be categorized into groups and the work prioritized.

Once the situational analysis is complete, planners typically proceed to detail an actual marketing plan with five sections:

1. *Assumptions:* Inclusion of a well-defined and thoroughly described list of assumptions ensures uniform understanding of the underlying premises.

2. *Mission, goals, and objectives:* These will complement and support those of the larger organization.

3. *Suggested strategies and options:* Each objective in the plan will have a strategy and a range of alternatives for accomplishing that end.

4. *Recommended strategic direction:* This is the major decision point and focuses on the future, including a broad statement of the plan's desired outcomes.

5. *List of recommended strategies and tactics:* Finally, the plan sets forth a more detailed description of who will do what within what timeline.

THE MARKETING BUDGET

Businesses budget for the promotion part of a marketing plan based on a percentage of sales revenue, what the business can afford, how much competitors seem to be spending, or what needs to be spent to accomplish the objectives. The latter method proves most applicable to libraries. All the budget elements will be detailed with a cost analysis, including personnel time, costs of user surveys, consultants, publicity, and the like.

MAKING STRATEGIC MARKETING DECISIONS

Implementing a successful marketing strategy entails several elements: conducting a marketing audit, identifying research tasks and using appropriate research techniques, and employing the marketing mix model.

The Marketing Audit

For many people, the term *audit* connotes something rather ponderous. The marketing audit need not be onerous but should be a regular part of the environmental assessment/situation analysis. "The marketing audit is a tool or process that enables a library to look at its audiences, services and products in light of current environmental influences," says Wakeley [29]. He provides checklists and suggestions and describes a case study. In the audit, staff members analyze each product or service in light of all others and look at alternatives. Action plans for each product and service are then developed. Olson offers another tool for audit purposes in the form of a list of questions that require the assessor to consider the library through the eyes of its clients [30].

Market Research Tasks

Market research is performed through four steps. In the first, the librarian conducts a market analysis. Librarians traditionally survey library users and nonusers, gathering information in as rigorous and systematic a manner as possible. Such essential information provides the background for decision making about everything from pricing to image projection.

In step two, the librarian considers the framework within which the library operates. If the librarian has done an environmental assessment as part of the situation analysis, there exists a good general picture. If the environment has not yet been scanned, one can gather information from secondary sources. For example, the librarian reviews major documents issued by the parent organization, such as a mission statement or strategic plan, and then looks at the literature to determine trends affecting the library and its users. These should include economic, political, and technological trends.

In the third stage, the librarian researches the competition. This step can also be done through secondary sources and gathering documents. Competitors can be either internal or external. *Internal competition* exists when departments in the organization vie for scarce resources. *External competition* may include other libraries, especially those with profit centers that sell their services, or vendors who market directly to users.

The fourth step seeks to stratify the market. *Market segmentation* is a process by which one categorizes market opportunities. User demographics are key. The library collects data on numbers of existing users, characteristics of the different professions served, and potential users. Because libraries cannot be all things to all people, decisions to limit or expand service necessitate hard data. Dragon notes that

> for too long the library has assumed that its market was every living human being in the community. This view has led libraries to offer too many hastily produced products for too few patrons. Effective libraries identify their market and offer products that will satisfy its needs [31].

Bunyan and Lutz illustrate this point by describing a hospital library's marketing effort targeted specifically at nurses. Librarians first performed an audit and user survey, then developed strategies to appeal to the nursing population, implemented their ideas, and evaluated the effect [32]. Cooper describes a similar effort to market hospital library services to attending physicians [33].

Demographic details drive important market segmentation variables. These include geography, profession, institutional affiliation, and age. In market research, demographics are augmented with psychographic variables, which include user wants, needs, and opinions such as the image of the library held by users and nonusers. Where demographic breakdowns are descriptive, psychographic ones show cause–effect relationships. A market segment can be defined by needs and desires and is based on information gathered through surveys or observation. Strategic design of products, services, and facilities benefits when the library management knows as much as possible about the user base. For example, if the library wishes to improve students' online search skills and knows that students need study space, the library could provide the space to entice them into greater contact.

Businesses find that technology allows them to tailor products, services, and media/promotion efforts to narrower target markets than ever before [34]. New technology delivers timely information to just those customers who will be interested. Libraries can devise similar technology-based strategies.

Market Research Techniques

Market research techniques generally identify user needs and then target products and services to meet those needs. They also assist in evaluating the impact and effectiveness of a marketing program. Research need not be so detailed and rigorous that it demands undue time or other resources. Librarians already have the skills necessary to do simple but meaningful market research.

Exploratory research helps identify problems and express research objectives. It establishes priorities for research and increases familiarity with the problem. Exploratory studies are flexible, meaning that researchers usually modify procedures as they proceed. The process often begins with a literature search on the problem area and involves a data-gathering step, such as an informal interview survey of key people. Descriptive research entails gathering and analyzing facts, and it requires "a clear specification of the who, what, when, where, why, and how of the research" [35]. It involves hypothesis testing and consequently is not as flexible as exploratory research.

Causal designs usually test relationship strength through some form of experiment. The investigator manipulates one or more independent variables and observes what happens to the dependent variable. Experiments can be done in a laboratory setting or in the field. Methods used in other social sciences are easily adapted to library settings. Simple regression and correlation and multiple regression are commonly used in marketing studies. Use of causal research may require outside assistance from consultants if the librarian's research skills and time are limited.

The user survey remains the most used method of gathering marketing information in libraries, whether through the use of written questionnaires or interview surveys. As one British writer expresses it, "User studies are on the whole a jolly good thing" [36]. They are useful for profiling the library's user population, identifying information needs, helping match resources to user needs, and monitoring the effectiveness of library service [37].

Focus groups provide another way to gain valuable information about user needs and desires. This group interview technique calls for a skilled moderator to ask open-ended questions and a discussion. One hospital library found that, although recruiting participants was a problem, "focus group interviews proved to be a useful, inexpensive way to obtain qualitative feedback about the library" [38]. See Chapter 7, The Application of Systematic Research, of this volume for a more detailed discussion of library research in general.

The Marketing Mix

To make strategic marketing decisions, the librarian uses a model for analyzing possible strategies in light of the information gathered through research. Although simplistic, the classic four *P*s—product, place, price, and promotion—offer a convenient framework for considering options. Politics has become a fifth *P* because of its importance and applicability in health sciences library settings.

Product/Service

A product is usually thought of as something tangible and a service as intangible. One could consider a mediated online search a mixture of both because the librarian has provided the expert service of negotiating the search strategy while a printed search product is subsequently handed to the customer. Answering a reference question is a service, while the library newsletter is a product. An evaluation of which products or services to winnow, which to continue, which to modify, and which new ones to offer can be assisted by knowledge of the product life cycle concept and a portfolio mix strategy.

Products and services typically follow a predictable course over time. Figure 4-1 depicts the introduction, growth, maturity, and decline stages of the product life cycle. Products differ in the length of time in each step and overall cycle. Likewise, individuals differ in their propensity to adopt innovative products and services. Figure 4-2 shows the common trend line for acceptance of innovation or, by extension, new products. During the introduction phase of the product life cycle, early adapters and innovators adopt a new idea. Strong sales and general acceptance of the product by the majority of users characterize the growth stage. Sales peak during the maturity stage, when a decision usually has to be made to revitalize the product or simply let it decline. Product sales decline in the last stage. If library services and support are tied to a product, such as a technology product, the product life cycle curves follow closely the pattern described in Figure 4-1 [39-40].

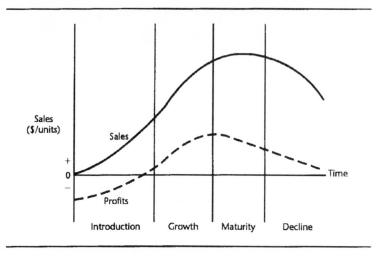

Figure 4-1: Product Life Cycle (From: Busch PS, Houston MJ. Marketing: strategic foundations. Homewood, IL: Irwin, 1985:412. Reprinted with permission.)

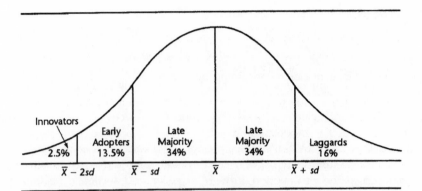

Figure 4-2: Diffusion of Innovations (From: Rogers EM. Diffusion of innovations. 4th ed. New York: Free Press, 1995: 262. Reprinted with permission.)

A company or library will have a group of products and services, each at different stages in the product life cycle. The portfolio mix model, first introduced by the Boston Consulting Group, helps in making decisions about whether to revitalize a product, let it be, or discontinue it [41]. The two-by-two matrix shown in Figure 4-3 plots market growth against market share. Products that no longer need heavy cash layouts for marketing but that still bring in profits

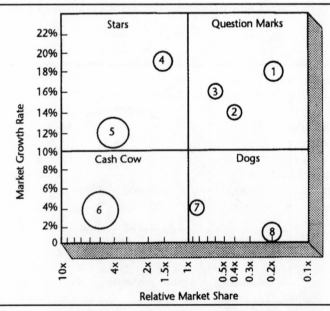

Figure 4-3: Boston Consulting Group's Market Share Index (From: Kotler P. Marketing management: analysis, planning, implementation, and control. 7th ed. Englewood Cliffs, NJ: Prentice Hall, 1991:39. Reprinted with permission.)

based on good reputations are called *cash cows* because the profits can be milked. *Rising stars* need cash for the introduction stage. *Dogs* are products that can be allowed to decline, and *question marks* are products with low growth and low market share [42]. By plotting library products and services this way, one can balance resource-consuming against resource-producing programs and services. Other portfolio mix theories supplement the BCG model.

Place

Place often includes distribution systems. In business, the transportation of goods and the arrangements made with distributors and other middlemen shape customers' perception. Efficient delivery of goods and services is equally important to the marketing of libraries where "barriers to distribution are spatial, temporal, physical, and perceptual" [43]. New information technology helps overcome spatial and temporal barriers. Phone, fax, and microcomputer capabilities greatly assist in providing outreach services within and outside the institution. Users in remote rural areas can now receive information just as quickly as do local faculty members. Lemkau, Burroughs, and LaRocco found that "electronic mail and facsimile transmission take on a new urgency when a library is marketing services to the community" [44]. Barriers are no longer just technological but also include cost and access considerations that are primarily organizational. Overcoming such barriers may become part of the library's marketing plan.

Pricing

Pricing poses difficult issues for most libraries. In the past, most or all services were offered at no charge, and costs were hidden from the end consumer. With the advent of photocopying and online searching, charges for library products and services became commonplace. Bell notes that "generally, librarians have been most concerned with the implications which fee-based services have for access to these services" [45].

From a marketing point of view, various pricing strategies can be exploited to either encourage or discourage use of services. While librarians dislike curtailment of services, strategic planning may point out that an expensive service necessitates charging full cost or at least a fair market price.

The pricing of electronic information poses even more complex problems. Arnold quips that

> setting the price for an electronic information product/service using traditional tools is like trying to repair an F-15 with a stone hammer. Information behaves differently from other products [46].

Companies in like circumstances use a variety of pricing strategies depending on the product life cycle and other factors. Libraries often do not know what it costs to produce one unit of a product or service. Knowing an average per-unit cost, which includes both fixed and variable components, can guide making pricing decisions.

Businesses often set a *skimming* policy for desirable new products. A high initial price will come down as the life cycle of the product plays out over time. Libraries might consider a skimming price strategy if a service must be rationed or demand must be kept low. Another new product strategy is *penetration pricing,* in which a low price introduces the product to a broad audience. The price may be increased after users have accepted the product [47].

Additionally, libraries can discount prices for prepaid accounts or other mechanisms that save staff time and effort. Libraries commonly pass through costs they are charged directly by others and subsidize indirect costs. When handling an interlibrary loan request for a client, for example, the library frequently absorbs internal processing costs, but any charges from the supplying library get passed to the requester. Fees or charges can be competition, cost, or demand oriented. Depending on the desired strategy, fees could be set equal to, higher than, or lower than those of competitors. In a cost orientation, a library decides if it wants to simply cover its costs, make a profit, or subsidize the service. In contrast, demand-oriented methods reflect what the user is willing to pay. In all cases, a mixture of elements is possible [48].

Promotion/Communication

Many people equate marketing with promotion and promotion with advertising. Promotional strategies include more than advertising and must be in balance with product, price, and place considerations. Bush and Houston define *promotional strategies* as "the set of activities that a firm employs to communicate to buyers in an attempt to stimulate their demand" [49]. Promotion can inform, persuade, and remind users about the library and its services.

Advertising is but one component of promotion and includes any paid form of communication that is not targeted to one individual. It usually includes television, radio, magazines, and newspapers. Individual health sciences libraries do not often use paid advertising, except perhaps for job ads in the mass media. However, newsletters and other publications such as brochures are forms of advertising libraries produce routinely. Personal selling is a second form of advertising and involves every face-to-face communication with a user.

Packaging is yet another form of promotion. "The promotional properties of a package derive mainly from the use of color, lettering, and illustrations" [50]. Viewed this way, libraries should pay close attention to every piece of documentation that comes from the library. How does the mediated online search look when the user gets it? Does a cover letter or form transmit a positive image of the library? How does the library's Web site look, and what image does it project?

Public relations activities seek to establish goodwill. These are not paid messages, although the staff time involved may entail a considerable cost. Publicity is a part of public relations, including any unpaid message that appears in the mass media such as press releases [51]. Other promotional strategies include contests, demonstrations, exhibits, and displays. Internet Web pages also have become increasingly important and expected parts of an institution's image.

Promotional messages must be well thought out and integrated with the overall marketing plan. What is the objective of the message? Does it define a target audience? Is the content clear? Is the style consistent with the intent? Is the format suitable? Evaluation of the impact of the library's strategy can be formal or informal, but it serves to guide future efforts.

Political

Although Kotler [52] adds both the words power and public relations to the traditional four *P*s of marketing, this chapter combines those two concepts under the term *politics.* Webster's *Ninth New Collegiate Dictionary* gives two definitions for the word *politics:* "competition between competing interest groups or individuals for power and leadership" and the "total complex of relations between people in society" [53]. Griffith believes that, in libraries, "marketing can be very effective in the political arena" [54]. In this realm the library administrator identifies decision makers who influence funding, targeting them for marketing and appropriate messages. "If the decision makers have been researched thoroughly, one should be able to determine their needs and be able to deal with them more productively" [55]. One should also identify the people who may not be in decision-making roles but who influence choices or act as opinion leaders.

HEALTH SCIENCES LIBRARY MARKETING STRATEGIES

Outlined here are six steps that health sciences library staff can use to develop and employ an effective marketing strategy.

Step One: Create an Integrated Marketing Effort

As mentioned earlier, all departments in the library have to participate in the marketing effort, not just public services departments. The best way to assure widespread commitment to the concept is to involve all library staff in the planning effort.

Step Two: Evaluate Innovative Management Techniques

Front-line staff hold the best ideas for new or revised products or services. By stimulating and rewarding new ideas, a climate for innovation becomes part of a library's culture. Relations with professionals outside the institution and an awareness of what is going on at other libraries promote innovation.

Step Three: Employ Multiple Promotion Efforts

Libraries enjoy many possible strategies for promotion. The mix of strategies will be individualized during the marketing planning process and will depend on target markets and objectives. Andreasen warns against the one-best-program approach, in which the "librarian decides on the best advertisement, the best poster, or the best brochure and uses it alone" [56]. One should experiment with different marketing strategies for different target markets and learn what a good mix can do. A combination of successes can work together for a positive payoff [57] and may include several techniques, described in the following sections.

Direct Mail or Phone

With word processors to help personally address and label letters, direct mail can be targeted at specific markets. Letters, memos, and postcards are effective direct communication tools [58]. Sending out unsolicited electronic mail to groups is not considered good etiquette. For blind contacts, print remains the more acceptable medium.

One study compared the effectiveness and efficiency of three promotional devices to introduce a new selective dissemination of information program at Ohio State University (OSU). An opinion leadership effort involved contacting individuals named by others as influential and describing to them a library service, then asking them to tell four colleagues about it. OSU also tried a blitz approach that included sending letters and following up with presentations at department meetings. A telephone solicitation approach used direct marketing, calling listed names. All three approaches proved equally effective, but the blitz and phone methods were less expensive and more efficient [59].

Group Activities

Cooperative marketing efforts can be a cost-effective and mutually beneficial way to promote services. Library cooperative networks can develop marketing plans and implement them with pooled resources. "Marketing can help more librarians move successfully from an institution-based business to a network-based business that will better serve individuals who need information" [60].

Advisory groups such as library committees are formed for many reasons, but they can be used as promotional tools if members are selected carefully for their "opinion leader" qualities as well as their interest in the library. Task forces and other ad hoc committees, such as IAIMS planning committees, can also play a role in promoting communication and understanding about the library. User groups are becoming more common, especially for microcomputer hardware and software support [61]. One institution targets intensive users who represent their departments and are given discounts on training and other special considerations in return for helping others in their work group. This takes some pressure off library staff and assures distributed expertise across the university. Software such as Majordomo can be used to set up chat rooms or areas on the Internet for sharing opinions. The library can act as a neutral sponsor in the organization and facilitate these group discussions.

Friends of the Library

"Friends groups are organized on a dues-paying membership basis for the purpose of promoting and supporting the library" [62]. They also do lobbying, promotion, and publicity; assist with programs and events; honor staff members with awards; and are "library promoters par excellence" [63]. See Chapter 2, Fiscal Management in Health Sciences Libraries, for a fuller discussion of the role of friends groups in fiscal management of the library.

While friends groups are usually thought of solely in terms of fund-raising, a survey about friends groups for medical rare book found that "friends groups play a much less significant role in providing money for acquisitions than oral tradition has led us to believe" [64]. Aside from fund-raising, friends groups perform other useful functions, such as public relations. Gilman warns, however, that the purpose and role must be clear and the library leadership must actively take part in the planning and ongoing maintenance of the group [65]; hence, it is advisable to compare the effort and the payback of such groups.

Publications

Virtually all libraries publish something: library guides, bibliographies, newsletters or columns in newsletters, reports, brochures, price lists, interlibrary loan or photocopy request forms, floor plans, journal cancellation or addition lists, notices on the Internet, or banners on database interfaces. The more publishing a library does, the more necessary it is to have expertise in designing the publications. A set of standards should be established concerning logo, message, format, and consistency. These guidelines apply equally to electronic publications and Web pages.

Administrative Writing

The astute library administrator will produce all reports, memos, and other communications in a professional manner. Electronic mail has increased the volume of communication, but standards of businesslike decorum are frequently lacking. Electronic mail also discourages a paper trail so that tracking becomes difficult. Gilman emphasizes two reports of particular importance:

> the budget request and the annual report. The former is perhaps the more important, as the institution's administration receives it just before it allocates funds for library operations [66].

Annual reports offer an opportunity to communicate about the library's accomplishments and enhance the image of the library and its staff.

Multimedia

Videotapes and slides continue to be useful promotion vehicles and orientation devices. Health sciences libraries find hypertext applications displayed on monitors at the library entrance useful for everything from floor plans to detailed descriptions of available services. Satellite technology allows one-way or two-way interactive video. The National Library of Medicine's information updates via two-way voice and one-way video are especially effective and informative. Libraries with outreach missions can effectively teach, promote, and interact with remote users via modern technology.

Mass Media

Press releases to newspapers and radio and television stations often yield widespread and free publicity. Most institutions screen press releases through a communications department to assure consistency and quality. The same department will usually help the library produce an appropriate release. It is to the library's advantage to keep that department up-to-date on library activities.

The fastest-growing source of popular mass media exposure is the Internet. Because the Internet is international, large numbers of people may view Web pages. Information provided on these pages should be appropriate for this wide and diverse audience.

Exhibits, Demonstrations, and Displays

Exhibits at the entrance of the library can introduce the patron to the facility and services. Exhibits in the library lobby seem less common in health sciences libraries than formerly, but they are more often done for promotion at conferences and meetings. That said, it remains that

> exhibits and demonstrations permit personal communication, the single most effective method of announcing the advantages of a service and stimulating desire

for it. Applicable in both are promotional pieces such as brochures, posters, and video or slide/tape productions on the services being marketed [67].

A display of book jackets for recently received titles is simple and effective. A kiosk with an interactive Web page not only is attractive but can assist the new patron in becoming oriented.

Several useful handbooks exist for detailed instructions on how to plan, organize, and technically produce an effective exhibit [68-72]. Libraries also can offer computer software demonstrations and live interactive sessions with online databases to attract users. For example, NLM encourages exhibits and demonstrations of PubMed, Internet Grateful Med, and MEDLINEPlus at professional medical meetings, with outstanding results. Also, state and regional medical library associations actively exhibit to end users. Individual libraries coordinate computer fairs that are increasingly popular with users. Such an annual event can be particularly effective in promoting recent or upcoming library computer services and can add names to your mailing lists.

Step Four: Provide Training for Library Users

Health sciences libraries routinely offer training to end users in online searching of various databases. This also presents the perfect opportunity to promote library services of all types. Usually when a user becomes an avid searcher, he or she appreciates the availability of a professional searcher for more comprehensive bibliographies. Searching always brings up the question of article availability and the opportunity to promote photocopy and interlibrary loan services or inform users that the library is their gateway to outside resources. The addition of full-text databases and access to publishers' Web pages for the very latest journal issues are increasingly popular and a tremendous benefit to users. Librarians must seize the opportunity to announce these offerings.

Step Five: Enhance Help Desks and Consumer Health Services

Larger libraries have become complex with the addition of computer labs, support for software and hardware, teleconferencing capabilities, and curricular involvement. Because this confuses even the seasoned user, more libraries are adopting a help desk or telephone support center. With such desks, libraries promote a phone number for information that includes more than traditional library information, primarily so users can be referred to the proper person or division in the organization. Numerous versions of this one-stop-shopping approach exist, and, as integrated information organizations proliferate, questions of cross training and scheduling and quality management will need to be further addressed. Each help desk interaction with a user leaves an impression of the library and contributes to a positive or negative image.

Many health sciences libraries welcome the general public. A hospital may offer a separate consumer health information library, telephone assistance, or mail services. The National Library of Medicine and Medical Library Association are becoming increasingly involved in extending consumer health information. Hospital and academic libraries with restricted physical access may offer services remotely; electronic and postal mail or facsimile transmission may be used to distribute materials. The library's Web page may link to patient materials.

Step Six: Train Library Staff in Customer Relations

Customers look for access, communication, competence, courtesy, credibility, reliability, responsiveness, security, tangibles, and evidence that the service supplier knows its customers [73]. In the commercial segment, customers can tell which retail businesses have hammered home a customer service philosophy. Library management should insist that objectives related to service quality be integrated into the strategic plan and, to increase staff understanding of the value of customer service from a marketing standpoint, establish quality management training programs for new and continuing staff.

ADDRESSING MARKETING ISSUES

Early in this chapter, seven marketing issues that challenge library administrators were set forth. These dilemmas will respond to the application of marketing theory and techniques in numerous ways.

1. *Does the library have too much business?* Target the library's market, define its products/services, and take the time to plan. When feeling overworked, it is especially hard to find planning time, yet it is imperative that boundaries be set so users and staff understand and share service expectations. A conscious decision may be made to accept more business but at the same time to lobby with administration for more dollar support based on the library's popularity. The price of certain services or products can either discourage business or make it profitable.
2. *Is the library restricted by a tradition of low pricing?* Reeducate users to place a higher value on information. This can be done as part of the marketing for the information literacy mission. As librarians train users to do some of their own bibliographic work, they can also explain and promote the value of mediated searching and other services available for a price. Just as the changing health care marketplace has made health care consumers more aware of the cost of care, the changing in-

formation marketplace offers new ways to increase awareness of the cost and value of information.

3. *Does the library face user expectation management problems?* Communicate realities via effective promotion efforts and persist in communicating them. This can be accomplished in a positive way by describing the situation and alternatives in a rational manner. Rather than complain, promote understanding.

4. *Is there a fee/free dichotomy?* Clarify the library's pricing policy. Understand the true cost of each product or service provided by the library. While the library may opt to subsidize some products and services and not others, the decisions should be made with as complete a set of decision tools as possible.

5. *Are market definition and outreach a problem?* Identify library markets, and go through the planning process. Once library decision makers discover the demographics of the present market, they are in a position to change them purposefully.

6. *Is marketing different for different kinds of libraries?* Yes, in some respects. A marketing plan differentiates each individual library and informs users of unique service offerings or restrictions.

7. *Is the library part of a larger integrated organization without a marketing orientation?* If the library markets successfully, it should serve as a model for the rest at the organization. This puts it in the advantageous position of being at the forefront, gathering data that will be useful to the larger organization.

Rolled together, these seven issues form a larger and essential question:

Do librarians have the will to live and thrive by competing, collaborating, and leading?. . . Do librarians know who they are? Do they know what they must do? And, Do they have the nerve [74]?

The answer is absolutely yes.

MARKETING SCENARIOS

The following fabricated scenarios illustrate two exercises in marketing health sciences libraries.

Academic Health Sciences Library

Once the planning group at Lakeside Health Sciences University agreed to put together an IAIMS planning grant proposal, members realized they needed to know more about campus users and, indeed, needed to develop a better idea of what information services were needed. They hired a graduate student to write a survey instrument, which was widely distributed. The results were heartening for the planning group because by and large the information services and technology units were highly regarded and enjoyed a positive image. Needs became evident for microcomputer support and training, better access to the electronic knowledge resources via the campus and hospital networks, and ease in moving from one network to the other.

In response, the group created a written document outlining planning steps and ways to let users know what would change. Because service image and use were already good, the main task was one of expectations management or communicating how things would be improved. By the time the proposal was written, most people on campus were aware of what IAIMS could mean to the institution and for them. Use of the marketing techniques had produced conditions favorable to the successful implementation of IAIMS.

Hospital Library

When Kathy Ferguson began working at River Falls Community Hospital, she made it a point to get to know her users better. In a one-person library, she had the chance to do everything, but she asked herself, "What should that everything be?"

In identifying her market, Kathy went outside the library and talked to people. She got a feel for who was already using the library, then she explored funding. She found that the medical staff provided most of the budget, primarily because the library committee chair was an influential opinion leader. The medical staff included some extremely heavy users but had a large number of nonusers. Nursing staff were fairly heavy users, but the education and administrative units were not. The library was located next to the medical staff lounge, but was in the basement and far from any major corridors or elevators.

Kathy devised a plan to reach her goal of better serving more users. She first targeted nonphysicians in her marketing plan and succeeded in relocating the library near the cafeteria and education department where there was a good deal of traffic. She attended medical staff meetings to update that group and be visible and started writing a monthly column in the hospital newsletter. She also targeted hospital administrators, sending them unsolicited notices of new material of interest to them. She befriended the leader of the hospital auxiliary and promoted the idea of providing patient education information to patients and the community. Use of marketing strategies produced a new, outgoing image of the library with greater potential for growth.

WHY TIME AND MONEY SHOULD BE SPENT ON MARKETING

"An assessment of the position of libraries today leads inescapably to the same conclusion: How can libraries afford not to market their services?" [75]. With other departments competing for resources, the library needs to keep a high profile. Although users need library services, the library itself needs users' support and the goodwill of all stakeholders. Marketing strategies have been used successfully in business organizations and increasingly in libraries [76], but they offer special advantages to health sciences libraries. According to Kotler, "there are three types of companies: those who make things happen, those who watch things happen, those who wonder what happened" [77]. Health sciences libraries hold an advantageous position in an era of rapid change. They are well situated to profit from the opportunities to market themselves and their services.

REFERENCES

1. Kotler P. Marketing management: analysis, planning, implementation, and control. 7th ed. Englewood Cliffs, NJ: Prentice Hall, 1991:18.

2. Ibid., 4.

3. McKenna R. Marketing is everything. Harv Bus Rev 1991 Jan/Feb;69(1):65-79.

4. Sherman S. Know your product, your competition, your clientele. In: Sherman S. ABC's of library promotion. 3rd ed. Metuchen NJ: Scarecrow, 1992:28.

5. Crawford W, Gorman M. Future libraries: dreams madness & reality. Chicago: American Library Association, 1995:7-8.

6. Kotler, op. cit., 4.

7. Wasserman P, Ford GT. Marketing and marketing research: what the library manager should learn. J Libr Admin 1980 Spring;1(1):19-29.

8. Weingard DE. Marketing for libraries and information agencies. Norwood, NJ: Ablex, 1984:55.

9. Kotler, op. cit., 8.

10. Senge PM. The fifth discipline: the art and practice of the learning organization. New York: Doubleday/Currency, 1990.

11. Cooper ER. Marketing the hospital library to physicians: one approach. Bull Med Libr Assoc 1991 Jan;79(1):86-7.

12. Bunyan LE, Lutz EM. Marketing the hospital library to nurses. Bull Med Libr Assoc 1991 Apr;79(2):223-5.

13. Wasserman, op. cit., 20.

14. Covell DG, Uman GC, Manning PR. Information needs in office practice: are they being met? Ann Intern Med 1985 Oct;103(4):596-9.

15. Gorman P, Ash J, Helfand M. Information needs and resources of rural and non-rural primary care physicians. Clin Res 1992;40:567A.

16. Gorman P, Ash J, Wykoff L. Can primary care physicians' questions be answered by using the medical literature? Bull Med Libr Assoc 1994 Apr;82(2):140-6.

17. Cihak H. Marketing CD-ROM and other electronic library services. Comput Libr 1997 Jun;17(6):73-6.

18. Fifteenth Anniversary Task Force, Library Instruction Round Table, American Library Association. Information for a new age: redefining the librarian. Englewood, CO: Libraries Unlimited, 1995:73.

19. White HS. Librarians and marketing. Libr J 1989 Aug;114(13):78-9.

20. McClure CR, Moen WE, Ryan J. Libraries and the Internet/NREN. Westport, CT: Mecklermedia, 1994.

21. Rummel KK, Pence E. Persuasive public relations for libraries. Chicago: American Library Association, 1983:15.

22. Leerburger BA. Marketing the library. White Plains, NY: Knowledge Industries Publications, 1982.

23. Sirkin AF. Marketing planning for maximum effectiveness. Spec Libr 1991 Winter;82(1):1-6.

24. St. Clair G. Marketing and promotion in today's special library. ASLIB Proc 1990 Jul/Aug;42(7/8):213.

25. Mueller-Alexander JM. Alternative sources for marketing research in libraries. Spec Libr 1991 Summer;82(3):159-64.

26. Crawford, op. cit.

27. Ash J, Beck JR. A systems approach to planning biomedical information services. In: Clayton P, ed. Assessing the value of medical informatics: 15th Annual Symposium on Computer Applications in Medical Care. New York: McGraw-Hill, 1992:481-5.

28. Sherman, op. cit., 217.

29. Wakeley, PJ. The marketing audit: a new perspective on library services and products. Bull Med Libr Assoc 1988 Oct;76(4):323-7.

30. Olson, CA. Test your library's marketing IQ. Med Ref Serv Q 1993 Fall;12(3):75-83.

31. Dragon AC. Marketing the library. Wilson Libr Bull 1979 Mar;53(7):498-502.

32. Bunyan LE, Lutz EM. Marketing the hospital library to nurses. Bull Med Libr Assoc 1991 Apr;79(2):223-5.

33. Cooper ER. Marketing the hospital library to physicians: one approach. Bull Med Libr Assoc 1991 Jan;79(1):86-7.

34. Webster FE. The changing role of marketing in the corporation. J Marketing 1992 Oct;56(4):1-17.

35. Churchill GA. Marketing research: methodological foundations. 4th ed. Chicago: Dryden Press, 1987:82.

36. Cronin B. Assessing user needs. ASLIB Proc 1981 Feb;33(2):37-47.

37. Ibid., 39-40.

38. Robbins K, Holst R. Hospital library evaluation using focus group interviews. Bull Med Libr Assoc 1990 Jul;78(3):311-3.

39. Wood EJ. Strategic marketing for libraries: a handbook. New York: Greenwood Press, 1988.

40. Potts G. Exploit your product's service life cycle. Harv Bus Rev 1988 Sep/Oct;66(5):32-6.

41. Wood, op. cit., 10-15.
42. Kotler, op. cit., 39.
43. Bell JA. Marketing reference services: translating selected concepts into action for a specific practice setting. In: Wood MS, ed. Cost analysis, cost recovery, marketing, and fee-based services: a guide for the health sciences librarian. New York: Haworth Press, 1985:137.
44. Lemkau HL Jr, Burrows S, La Rocco A. Marketing information services outside the medical center. In: Wood MS, ed. Cost analysis, cost recovery, marketing, and fee-based services: a guide for the health sciences librarian. New York. Haworth Press, 1985:155.
45. Bell, op. cit., 146.
46. Arnold SE. Marketing electronic information: theory, practice, and challenges 1980-1990. In: Williams ME, ed. Annual review of information science and technology. New York: Elsevier, 1990:113.
47. Busch PS, Houston MJ. Marketing: strategic foundations. Homewood, IL: Richard D. Irwin, 1985:565-70.
48. Kotler P, Bloom PN. Marketing professional services. Englewood Cliffs, NJ: Prentice Hall, 1984.
49. Busch, op. cit., 622.
50. Ibid., 627.
51. Ibid., 629.
52. Kotler P. Megamarketing. Harv Bus Rev 1986 Mar/Apr;64(2):117-24.
53. Webster's ninth new collegiate dictionary. Optical laser disc. Falls Church, VA: Highlighted Data, 1992.
54. Griffith, LM. Political marketing of the rural library. Wilson Lib Bull 1989 May;63(9):44-7.
55. Ibid., 45.
56. Andreasen AR. Advancing library marketing. J Libr Admin 1980 Fall;1(3):17-32.
57. Muir, RF. Marketing your library or information service to business. Online 1993 Jul;17(4):41-6.
58. Kohn R, Tepper K. You can do it: a PR skills manual for libraries. Metuchen, NJ: Scarecrow, 1981.
59. Stern LW, Craig CS, La Greca AJ, Lazorick GJ. Promotion of information services: an evaluation of alternative approaches. J Am Soc for Info Science 1973 May-Jun;24(3):171-8.
60. Moulton BL. Marketing and library cooperatives. Wilson Libr Bull 1981 Jan;55(5):347-352.
61. Gilman NJ. Administration: promoting and enhancing the library program. In: Darling L, Colaianni LA, Bishop D, eds. Handbook of medical library practice. 4th ed. v. 2. Chicago: Medical Library Association, 1988:359-60.
62. Edsall MS. Library promotion handbook. Phoenix: Oryx Press, 1980:185.
63. Ibid., 186.
64. Mueller MH, Overmeier JA. An examination of characteristics related to success of friends groups in medical school rare book libraries. Bull Med Libr Assoc 1981 Jan;69(1):9-13.
65. Gilman, op. cit., 360.
66. Ibid., 363.

67. Lemkau op. cit., 154.

68. Leerburger, op. cit.

69. Edsall, op. cit.

70. Schaeffer M. Library displays handbook. New York: Wilson, 1991.

71. Coplan K. Effective library exhibits: how to prepare and promote good displays. New York: Oceana, 1958.

72. Garvey M. Library displays: their purpose, construction and use. New York: Wilson, 1969.

73. Kotler, Marketing management, op. cit., 464.

74. McClure, op. cit., 367

75. Edinger JA. Marketing library services: strategy for survival. Coll Res Libr 1980 July; 41(4):328-32.

76. Tucci VK. Information marketing for libraries. In: Williams ME, ed. Annual review of information science and technology. New York: Elsevier, 1988: 59-82.

77. Kotler, Marketing Management, op. cit., 32.

5

The Technological Transformation of Health Sciences Libraries

Audrey Powderly Newcomer

Technology is transforming libraries. Today's library cannot thrive without fundamentally changing in response to the infusion of new computing, instructional, and communication technologies. These factors alter not only the operation of libraries; they also transform the library's function within the parent organization. The value of the library no longer derives from what it holds but from what it can do. Reflecting on the infusion of these technologies, changing paradigms, the human dimension, and associated costs, library administrators must formulate a clear vision of both the larger environment and the role they play within it to manage an ongoing transformation successfully.

Effective library administrators know the environment in which they operate. They plan within the context of a known environment to establish an active and dynamic library presence. Health sciences librarians encounter both the challenges facing general academic libraries and those confronting health care. In the information era, all libraries grapple with factors such as journal pricing, copyright, electronic publishing and licensing, full-text materials, the fluid nature of the Internet, and the growth of intranets. Within health sciences libraries, information issues related to health care (e.g., medical informatics, hospital accreditation, patient education, renewed curriculum, competitive research, and limited funding) demand active and prompt response. Braude has used the metaphor of natural selection to demonstrate that the position of health sciences librarians has in the past been shaped by events in the environment [1]. Their willingness to change enabled librarians to respond to these events in an effective manner.

In addition, effective library administrators enlarge the scope of planning and service development so as to customize and integrate libraries into the larger organization. By focusing attention on programs that are necessary for the organization to meet its business strategy, libraries become essential. In the migration away from owning traditional resources and making documents available, the library will feature access to new digital resources and a renewed service orientation. As the focus shifts from the simple provision of information to the development of knowledge and customization of services to satisfy user needs, libraries will become a value-added service.

In the 1980s, Matheson envisioned that libraries could demonstrate their preeminence as the organization that knows how to locate and mine knowledge [2]. Today, technological progress assists the profession in identifying and staking out new roles and alliances valuable to institutions and individuals while maximizing the strengths and skills of librarians. With modern technology, any user can find more information than can be utilized in a lifetime, and responsive librarians enlarge their participation by moving from a role of supporter to that of collaborator. In this context, supporting is "doing for others," whereas collaborating is "working with others." Enriched by cooperation with additional partners, librarians can expand their sphere of influence at the institutional level.

Effective library administrators also use outcome measures and practice evidence-based librarianship to demonstrate accountability. Now, more than ever, library administrators must clearly articulate goals and devise methods for measuring outcome. Anderson draws a parallel between evidence-based medicine and the need for evidence-based librarianship to identify and correct gaps in the professional knowledge base [3]. By evaluating services rather than processes, gaps in knowledge can be identified and librarians remain responsive to rapid changes in expectations and needs. For example, given the goal to elevate the searching capabilities of health professionals, one would measure the content retained after a training session rather than the number of sessions taught. It shouldn't be collection size but what libraries do that plays the most important factor in accreditation and institutional ranking decisions. How libraries demonstrate the impact of their contributions will determine whether this is indeed the case. As Braude so aptly summarizes, research begins with a question and ends with a publication, only to reinitiate the entire process [4].

Legacy-based thinking must be reshaped in the face of new realities. For instance, it is unrealistic to assume that all health sciences library services can be subsidized or that the library can be all things to all people. Instead library administrators must make choices within the harsh light of economics by assessing institutional needs and revamping services accordingly. Health information professionals must invest in change and become change agents. By providing administrators with meaningful data in support of enterprise-wide information policy and resource allocation decisions, fiscal accountability is demonstrated and the awareness of library contributions heightened. Furthermore, effective library administrators uphold a professional code of ethics. As Peay noted in his 1998 Janet Doe lecture, a major factor that distinguishes health sciences librarians from other information specialties is a formal professional code of ethics [5]. The introduction to the Medical Library Association's (MLA) Code of Ethics for Health Sciences Librarianship establishes a vital perspective: "The health sciences librarian believes that knowledge is the sine qua non of informed decisions in health care, education and research and the health sciences librarian serves society, clients and the institution, by working to ensure that informed decisions can be made" [6]. The code serves as a touchstone for decisions and a measure for success.

Finally, effective library administrators promote and practice life-long learning. Health sciences librarians have a rich history of promoting life-long learning for their users. Decades ago Brodman admonished librarians to educate for a generation hence instead of for the problems of today, so that health information professionals would not perform tomorrow's tasks with yesterday's concepts [7]. Life-long learning develops the ability to make projections and transitions. By regularly renewing the knowledge base, responsiveness to information needs can be achieved within a volatile environment. In a time of fundamental change, library administrators must seek out creative means to support and upgrade the skills and knowledge base of both users and staff.

It is within this framework that the impact of technology on the administration of the health sciences library is discussed. This chapter should be construed not as a comprehensive treatise but rather as a broad overview of several areas of technology that previously altered and continue to influence the decisions of library administrators.

INFUSION OF TECHNOLOGY INTO LIBRARIES

Health sciences librarians have consistently led in the application of technology, covering a tremendous scope of activities, from routine library applications to health care informatics. Changing technology demanded new responses from librarians and other health information professionals. The infusion of technology produced simple incremental change but also spawned a paradigm shift. Tapscott and Caston state that "a paradigm is a set of rules and regulations that establish or define boundaries and dictate how to behave within these boundaries in order to be successful" [8]. Consequently, a "paradigm shift is the change to a new set of rules." For example, in the military, cell phones have replaced walkie-talkies. In educational media, slides are being replaced by presentation software. Within librarianship, the World

Wide Web represents the biggest technological impact on libraries perhaps since the assimilation of photocopy machines in the 1950s.

When, as a result of a change or discovery, the existing paradigm comes into conflict with a new reality, a different paradigm tends to emerge, one that helps create a new way of seeing the world. In addition, it generally provides a new vocabulary, such as the use of the term *health information professional* in lieu of *librarian*. As new paradigms develop, they do not necessarily replace the old paradigm but may have an independent parallel existence. This chapter offers a basic overview of paradigm shift resulting from the evolution of library automation. The discussion is intended as a point of departure for later discussion of the continuing changes in the dynamic environment in which libraries operate. For other relevant reviews, the reader may refer to Pizer's review of technology [9] or Bunting's general review of the field [10].

This chapter's overview begins with the first efforts to automate library functions and includes the infusion of technology in libraries through the 1970s. These efforts largely benefited staff and only indirectly benefited users. The chronological commentary progresses to a "second generation" of library automation in the 1980s. These efforts concentrated on the integration and interdependence of the modules of online service that provide end users greater access to information. It was only during the 1990s, a "third generation" of technology, that the focus shifted to the interdependence of library systems with external systems. This most recent set of developments has had tremendous impact on users and has prompted new services, roles, and relationships.

First Generation: Library and Other Technology in the 1970s

The modern Internet began as an extension of a computer network originally formed in the United States during the 1960s by the Advanced Research Projects Agency (ARPA). Working under contract to the U.S. Department of Defense, ARPA initially connected computers at the Stanford Research Institute in California, the University of California at Los Angeles (UCLA), the University of California at Santa Barbara (UCSB), and the University of Utah. This original linkage, the very first computer network, was called ARPANET (ARPA NETwork). Scientists built ARPANET to attain a network that would be able to function efficiently if part of the network was damaged. This concept was important to military organizations, which sought to maintain a working communications network in the event of nuclear war [11].

As ARPANET grew in the 1970s, and as more universities and institutions connected to it, users found it necessary to establish standards for the way data was transmitted over the network. To meet the needs of data transmission standards, computer scientists developed the Transmission Control Protocol (TCP) and the Internet Protocol (IP). During this period, various government, scientific, and academic groups developed their own networks (e.g., the Department of Energy's [DOE] Magnetic Fusion Energy Network [MFENet], the High Energy Physics NETwork [HEPNET], and the National Science Foundation NETwork [NSFNET]), and telecommunication standards became more critical [12].

In the 1970s, technology became firmly implanted in both hospital and academic medical center libraries. One of the most significant early developments was the automation of *Index Medicus*. For decades, reference librarians had searched and assisted patrons in searching for material in the printed indexes. The computerization of *Index Medicus* resulted in the premier biomedical database, MEDLINE. This online resource, developed by the National Library of Medicine (NLM), began coverage with 1966 and contained approximately ten million references to journal articles by 1999. It was supplemented by OLDMEDLINE, which contained an additional 771,287 citations indexed between 1960 and 1965 [13].

When online indexes first appeared, they were accessed by "dumb" terminals with acoustic telephone couplers and were largely a tool for librarians. At the time, NLM actively discouraged nonlibrarians from searching because it was considered impractical for most users to learn the exacting query protocols. Consequently, end users relied on a trained librarian intermediary to perform searches. In 1976, Bibliographic Retrieval Systems (BRS) began providing commercial online search services of MEDLINE. A host of competitors followed. Even after online searching became much easier due to improved software, end user searching did not increase dramatically until hardware improved. A significant advance in the searching interest and skills of users was not witnessed until the arrival of the personal computer.

Because of the high usage of serials in medical libraries, the tracking of serials and their contents became a prime target for automation. PHILSOM (Periodicals Holdings in Libraries of Schools of Medicine) provided an early system for the automated tracking of serials data [14].

Resources not located at a home library could be obtained by borrowing materials from other libraries through the process of interlibrary loan (ILL), and the volume of manual ILL transactions grew rapidly in the 1970s. Books were shipped between libraries, as were journal volumes until the advent of the inexpensive and reliable photocopier made it possible to send photocopies of the requested article instead. Photocopy technology created a paradigm shift, enlarging the activity of simple ILL to include the concept of one-way document delivery. Still, ILL continued to be the preferred term for obtaining photocopies or electronic transmissions from other libraries.

Online catalogs first became a reality in this era, building on the full MARC (Machine-Readable Cataloging) record planned and developed at the Library of Congress by Henriette Avram in the 1960s [15]. OCLC (Online Computer

Library Center) and a consortium of the country's research libraries (the Research Libraries Group) became the primary providers of automated cataloging on a national level. Each possessed enormous databases of bibliographic records and the ability to provide archival cataloging tapes of the records of a member library [16]. Early system developers recognized that the juxtaposition of the bibliographic record developed from the archival cataloging tapes and the item-level information typically found in the circulation record offered users a potential value-added product, the prototype for today's online catalog.

The first online public access catalogs (OPAC) started in the late 1970s with the simple objective of replicating existing library functions to make them more efficient and effective. Developers were sensitive to improving access without creating unnecessarily high learning curves for the traditional user accustomed to searching the traditional card catalog. Early adapters of online catalogs in health sciences libraries focused on three options. The first alternative was to turn to the commercial vendors of online circulation systems, such as CLSI or Dataphase, which promised to enhance these basic circulation systems to provide a rudimentary online catalog. Because most commercial systems were too expensive for small libraries to acquire independently, a number of libraries often collaborated with larger libraries to acquire a commercial system jointly.

A second option was to work with a larger library to develop a local union catalog, such as the MELVYL system at the University of California [17]. A select few were able to elicit the support of a computing services department to design their own system. These libraries then made their systems available to other libraries, creating a third option. Health sciences libraries without the computing resources to develop a local online system or the financial capital required for purchase of a commercial system could obtain a system developed by and for health sciences libraries.

The BACS (Bibliographic Access and Control System) system at Washington University School of Medicine [18] and the LIS (Library Information System) system at Georgetown University [19] enabled libraries to automate their local processes and were subsequently marketed to other libraries. These systems were less costly than their larger counterparts, focused on issues of primary concern to medical libraries, and could provide more customized approaches to user problems due to a much smaller customer base. All OPAC systems in the 1970s used proprietary languages and terminals hardwired to the system. Although these systems did improve the efficiencies and effectiveness of libraries, there is no evidence that these systems lowered the cost of operating libraries.

Parallel to the development of technology internal to libraries, the application of computer and information technology to biomedical endeavors created an entirely new discipline, medical informatics. Bloise and Shortliffe define *medical informatics* as "the rapidly developing scientific field that deals with the storage, retrieval, and optimal use of biomedical information, data, and knowledge for problem solving and decision-making" [20]. In the 1970s, this new discipline emerged from five separate fields: signal processing, database design, decision making, modeling and simulation, and natural language recognition [21].

Signal processing was used to develop computer algorithms to recognize and classify patterns automatically, such as in the electrocardiogram. Databases were built by designing and building systems that allowed one person to store information so that someone else could retrieve it without having to know the technical details about how the data was stored. Medical informatics facilitated decision-making processes by restructuring information based on the analysis of an expert and the creation of a computer-based model. The use of models and simulation provided a basis for planning, extrapolation beyond current experience, and sensitivity analysis. Finally, pursuit of a human–machine interface led to work on natural language recognition, and medical informaticists began to explore the confluence of these five subject areas.

Second Generation: Technology in the 1980s

The growing widespread use of the personal computer generated greater user expectations for computer systems of all kinds, but automated systems and products existed in isolation from each other. IBM held a monopoly on administrative applications. The MUMPS programming language was dominant in the clinical realm. Most educational software development was written for the Apple Macintosh platform. In the early 1980s, word-processing programs, database programs, spreadsheets, facsimile (fax) machines, and campus email systems became prevalent. By the middle of this period, the value of the personal computer increased significantly and moved from data processing to encompass the realm of communications as well.

Library computerization concentrated on the integration and interdependence of online modules. The ever-increasing demand for materials from the collections of academic libraries prompted the development of an ILL system that allowed libraries to establish a balance of trade for borrowing and lending. In the 1980s, the Midcontinental Region of the NLM's Regional Medical Library Program built a prototype ILL system, Octanet [22-23], based on the PHILSOM system. PHILSOM included the journal holdings of many participating libraries. Octanet's software included tables to establish the order in which a loan request should be sent to libraries owning the material. This capability allowed for a more equitable distribution of requests for materials among participating libraries.

Octanet served as the precursor for DOCLINE, NLM's automated ILL request and referral system. Many health sciences libraries relied on DOCLINE to secure copies of articles in the journal literature while using the ILL module of OCLC for borrowing books. The combined use of these two systems allowed health sciences libraries to more easily monitor the balance of trade and make adjustments. Additional commercial software programs, such as QuickDoc [24], enabled staff in ILL departments to manage increasing traffic in borrowing and lending. QuickDoc, a DOS-based program designed to interface with DOCLINE, allowed the ILL staff to automate record keeping and generate reports for all ILL activity regardless of the physical format of the actual request. The burgeoning reliance on the fax machine in the late 1980s allowed libraries to easily send copies of articles to another location. Initially many libraries reserved using the fax for articles needed for immediate clinical care because faxing was outside the regular work flow and increased the average amount of time to fill a request.

NLM's Grateful Med version of MEDLINE was introduced in 1986. It quickly became the focus of the majority of outreach efforts promoting current medical information directly to health professionals not affiliated with an institution having a medical library. The regional medical library program elicited the support of both academic and hospital libraries to market this system to health professionals nationwide. Other end user–assisted software for MEDLINE searching also emerged. Some examples of these products were PaperChase, CD+ (later OVID Technologies), and Knowledge Finder. The Pacific Southwest Regional Medical Library Service directly participated in the development of a Grateful Med document delivery counterpart, Loansome Doc, which was announced in 1989. The Loansome Doc software enabled users not otherwise affiliated with a health sciences library to make standing arrangements to receive articles from a designated library.

In early 1987, NLM signed its first experimental CD-ROM agreement with Cambridge Scientific Abstracts to use this new technology for accessing the MEDLINE database with cheaper, simpler search software. Eight competing commercial systems appeared by the following year. In 1988, NLM conducted a collaborative evaluation project to review CD-ROM system products at twenty-one locations [25]. These commercial vendors had enhanced the MEDLINE database with many value-added features. For example, while the NLM version used abbreviated titles, other vendors included the full title to eliminate confusion. Options to restrict search results to a library's local holdings were included. Most vendors created a search engine capable of querying MEDLINE and other similar databases without the need to rekey a search. With the later migration of reference databases from CD-ROM to client–server applications, users subsequently enjoyed more features and a further reduction in the amount of time needed to find information.

The second generation OPACs of the 1980s represented a dramatic step forward for bibliographic control. These systems advanced from circulation systems with add-on modules to truly integrated, value-added products. The second-generation online catalog was envisioned to represent a complete reference for all materials held by the library, from archives to computer-assisted instruction software programs. A noticeable trend in OPAC development was the movement from the proprietary systems of the 1970s to open system architecture in which proprietary hardware and software were not impediments to performance or system migration.

Libraries increasingly moved to integrated library systems. The decentralization of computing in the 1980s pushed system developers toward delivery of information at the end user's workstation. This outcome prompted the upgrading of dumb terminals to microcomputers to increase functionality and provide connectivity both from on campus and over the Internet. The provision of access from multiple platforms using seamless interfaces generated a great deal of discussion among vendors, libraries, and a wide variety of units within campus systems.

One hallmark of the 1980s was the transformation of the reference librarian from searcher to educator in both hospital and academic health sciences libraries. The academic health sciences librarian's role as educator expanded, with the greater involvement in curriculum-based instruction. Librarians worked with discipline-based faculty to teach sections of formal required courses. Hospital librarians working in both teaching and nonteaching hospitals offered a wide variety of online training programs. These programs paralleled the offerings in academic health sciences libraries varying from one-on-one sessions to classroom training and distance-based education.

The 1984 General Professional Education for Physicians (GPEP) report of the Association of American Medical Colleges (AAMC) recognized the impact of technology on physician education [26]. This report recommended that graduates be able to retrieve information from the published knowledge base, be able to analyze and correlate data about patients, and have a basic familiarity with computer technology. It further described mastery of several levels of increasingly complex computer skills, including using word processing and email, selecting and using educational materials, accessing databases, and evaluating systems, and the skills to use specialized systems and databases. The proposed instructional strategies for inculcating knowledge and skills included freestanding courses offered by the library, electives in medical informatics offered during the four years of medical education, and integrated informatics experiences within courses already in the formal required curriculum [27]. Further guidance on the inclusion of medical informatics in the curricula emerged in early 1999.

Many audiovisual departments within health sciences libraries were expanded to include educational software in support of the curriculum. Computer-assisted instruction included educational, administrative, and clinical applications. Commercially available medical decision support software (e.g., Iliad and QMR), full-text references (e.g., STAT-Ref and M.D. Consult), and informational updates (e.g., Clinical Alerts and American Medical News) were added to the library's collection of resources and available via the OPAC. Access to these materials, albeit used primarily by early adopters, was considered so vital that many libraries continued to produce printed lists or developed databases to provide supplemental information that was not included in the OPAC. This added a new dimension to course development in schools of medicine.

Information access in medical centers in the 1980s was characterized by a multiplicity of information systems, data and communications protocols, and hardware configurations. Concurrent with the birth of library information systems and document preparation software was the development of a myriad of other systems. Clinical information systems included clinical and ambulatory care medical records. Financial information systems included health care billing and grant management data. The need to integrate these three distinct enterprises within the infrastructure of networks, email, software support services, and specialized computing resources was soon apparent [28].

NLM emphasized the synergy between medical librarianship and medical informatics by funding informatics training programs and integrated academic/advanced information management systems initiatives [29]. This led to the development of the concept of an Integrated Advanced Information Management System (IAIMS). The primary focus of the IAIMS was to integrate electronic information from a wide array of sources and place this information at the fingertips of clinicians, researchers, and administrators to support their work. In 1984, NLM began providing grant assistance to medical centers, health sciences institutions, and other organizations eager to pursue the IAIMS vision.

In the 1980s, the pace of incorporating technology into the health care environment quickened. Rapid advances were made in health sciences libraries. Similar advances were being made in the growing field of informatics [30]. Both fields faced growing sophistication in their clientele, emphasized the delivery of relevant information, and were concerned with the production of new knowledge. Electronic biomedical information needed to be retrieved from and integrated into a variety of sources. Researchers and health professionals found that each system used idiosyncratic terminology that was not well correlated with other automated systems.

In this era, both health care and library practitioners envisioned a future with widespread access to more powerful, less expensive computers, improved telecommunications, and a huge array of diverse machine-readable biomedical information sources. Health professionals and researchers expected to be able to obtain information relevant to practice or research decisions when and where needed. This vision, however, could only be realized if automated systems could interpret their inquiries correctly, identify databases likely to have information relevant to these inquiries, and retrieve the pertinent information from those sources. In 1986, NLM began a long-term research and development project to build a Unified Medical Language System (UMLS). The UMLS project set out to design knowledge sources that could be used by computer programs to overcome the barriers to effective information retrieval caused by disparities in language and by the scattering of information across many databases and systems [31].

In 1987, the Association of Academic Health Sciences Library Directors (AAHSLD), a member of the Council of Academic Societies of the AAMC, conducted a survey. The survey attempted to identify the library systems or vendors being used for library operations, ascertain end user systems being used or contemplated, and measure the involvement of academic health sciences libraries with local area networks [32]. Early on, librarians recognized that despite the substantial value gleaned from bibliographic systems, bibliographic citations and abstracts were not sufficient to satisfy users. The search was not complete until the user could have access to the actual content online.

The Medical Informatics Section (MIS) of the Medical Library Association was established in 1988. Its primary purpose was to provide a platform for interaction and communication between medical librarians and professionals in the information and computer sciences working on projects of mutual interest. Members of the MIS participated at annual meetings, programs, cosponsored symposia, and informal discussions with other groups. An electronic newsletter bridged the communication gap between meetings. In January 1989, the journal *Academic Medicine* started a regular column on medical informatics.

This was the same year English computer scientist Timothy Berners-Lee introduced the concept of the Web [33]. Berners-Lee initially designed the Web to aid communication between physicists who were working in different parts of the world. He created a system of interconnected information on the Internet with browser software (e.g., Mosaic, Netscape Navigator, and Internet Explorer) to enable a computer to display pages of content. Various search engines emerged to provide assistance in searching specific topics. AltaVista, Yahoo!, Lycos, Excite, and other search engines assisted the user in finding information on the Web.

Third Generation: Accelerated Technological Change in the 1990s

By the 1990s, new technologies had dramatically changed the practice of medicine and the practice of health sciences librarianship. It was apparent that the pace of infusion of technology into health sciences libraries was accelerating. Increasing numbers of health professionals began to use the Internet, due in large part to the ability of the Web to easily handle multimedia documents. During this decade, the world witnessed the arrival and rapid disappearance of Gopher as one short-lived application of technology.

Gophers represented an extension to traditional in-house resources. These home-grown systems allowed access to both text and graphics as menu-based information. Any Gopher or wide area information system (WAIS) available to the user could then be included in an online catalog of resources. Over the course of a few years, Gophers and affiliated software were largely replaced by hypertext links to audio, video, and other resources offered through the Web. Hypertext consisted of an interlinked system of documents that allowed a user to move from one document to another in a nonlinear, associative way. Despite their short life, Gophers effectively demonstrated the concept of integrating outside resources into the library online catalog.

While electronic mail enabled basic electronic correspondence, the electronic discussion list provided a venue for multiple users to communicate with each other over an extended period of time. The power of collaboration was demonstrated in health sciences libraries through the use of email and email discussion lists. The AAHSL Electronic Discussion Group, begun in April 1989, was open only to members of the Association of Academic Health Sciences Libraries. This discussion group provided a forum for comment, opinion, questions, and information of interest. MEDLIB-L was a discussion list, begun in January 1991, that significantly increased the sharing of health sciences information across institutions nationwide [34]. Health sciences librarians could obtain input on an issue from a multitude of fellow professionals by sending one message to a single list address. Newsgroups provided an option to follow threads of messages and responses. The ability to send messages soon prompted the desire to send files.

In 1991, the staff of the Research Libraries Group developed Ariel software to digitize an article rather than simply photocopying it. Ariel increased transmission speed threefold and sent a potentially better quality document than fax technology, but it required a microcomputer at each end [35]. Consortia as well as libraries with collections in several locations found Ariel particularly helpful to forward materials from one location to another without physically moving the original item. Early Ariel versions generally required more staff time to operate because, unlike a regular fax, one could not see exactly what was sent. This resulted in instances of transmitting images a second time, thereby increasing the unit transaction cost.

NLM developed DocView in 1996 to deliver the digitized content of an article directly to the desktop computer of the end user. This software allowed the article to be electronically manipulated and the information to be integrated into application software on the health professional's desktop. Document delivery had thus shifted to information delivery. Off-site end users in particular appreciated this functionality. DocView represented yet another example of the incorporation of technology in libraries to meet the growing expectations of the end user. Products such as Ariel and DocView shortened the gap between the identification of a citation and the actual delivery of the full content.

With the growing number of online databases, end users have been exposed to a wider variety of resources. This increased exposure to information, paralleled with the inability of library budgets to keep pace with rising serial costs, shifted the emphasis from information ownership to access in the 1990s. One result was the creation of a market for commercial distribution centers. The CARL UnCover service [36], created in 1993 and later sold by the Colorado Alliance of Research Libraries, provided a commercial option for the already overtaxed ILL staff to obtain articles rapidly.

During this period, commercial vendors continued to sell library systems with increasingly more user-friendly interfaces using client server applications and a local area network. The number of electronic bibliographic databases increased beyond MEDLINE to include CINAHL (Cumulative Index to Nursing & Allied Health Literature) and PsycInfo as well as more specialized databases, such as Health Planning and Administration, Micromedex, International Pharmaceutical Abstracts, Bioethicsline, and many others. Current awareness services, such as Current Contents and Reference Update, closed the time lag between indexing and availability of information about an article. Some products allowed the user to further eliminate references already viewed in MEDLINE when performing a parallel search. Others provided the option to restrict search results to items available electronically in full text.

One clear impact of the proliferation of databases was an expansion of the health sciences librarian's role in teaching. Enhanced database search software continued to challenge infrequent searchers, and bibliographic instruction expanded. Instruction commonly differentiated between using a fixed vocabulary and less precise keyword searching. It also contrasted searching of a bibliographic file with queries of a full-text database. Introduction to literature searching, electronic resources, problem-based resources, email, the Web, and consumer education were incorporated into the formal curriculum of some schools in response to a report of the AAMC's Medical School Objectives Project [37].

Following the growth of client–server applications came a number of "free" MEDLINE sites available on the Web. Examples included America Online, Avicenna, HealthGate, Medscape, and Physicians Online. In June 1997, the NLM announced free Internet access to MEDLINE through either PubMed or Internet Grateful Med. PubMed was developed to provide user-directed, command-driven searching. It allowed a user to click on a citation with an embedded link to the full text of the article at a publisher's Web site. In contrast, Internet Grateful Med used the UMLS and was designed to simplify searching for infrequent users.

As of early 1999, searchers were noting deficiencies in NLM's unsophisticated search interface. Improvements were made, such as the ability to request related articles. Other MEDLINE vendors, particularly Ovid and SilverPlatter, remained viable because they offered tangible value-added benefits. Yet, what the free Web-based interfaces lacked in sophistication, they made up in ease of access, enormous potential for full-text access, and greater currency. Because the differing versions of MEDLINE search interfaces resulted in different search results, librarians were called on to educate their users about the reasons for these divergences and how to maximize search potential.

The 1990s brought parallel technological changes to health care providers. Evidence-based health care arose as a process for systematically finding, appraising, and using contemporaneous research findings as the basis for making clinical decisions. Sackett places things in perspective by stating that evidence-based medicine "builds on and reinforces but never replaces clinical skills, clinical judgement and clinical experience" [38]. The major barriers to implementing evidence-based health care include the sheer size of the medical literature, the lack of precise MEDLINE indexing for systematic reviews, and the multiplicity of studies and results on the same clinical question. It is also difficult to locate unpublished trials and relegate enough time to read and appraise the literature. However, this situation is slowly changing. While health professionals primarily relied on pharmaceutical representatives and traditional review articles in an earlier period, new sources of information became available. Many health sciences librarians embraced evidence-based practice and acquired subscriptions to supporting resources. The Cochrane Library became one respected resource to assist the practitioner in translating research into practice.

The Cochrane Collaboration is a worldwide voluntary group of health care providers, scientists, and consumers engaged in a collaborative effort to prepare, maintain and disseminate up-to-date systematic reviews of randomized controlled trials. This is important because the scientific community views randomized trial as the "gold standard" for judging the efficacy of a treatment modality. The systematic review process identifies all possible relevant evidence, both published and unpublished; selects studies using explicit inclusion criteria; synthesizes the results of multiple primary investigations; and interprets the clinical implications of the findings. If the data are statistically combined, the review is called a *quantitative review* or *meta-analysis*. In evidence-based care, one looks for the best external evidence to answer a clinical question, which is greatly enhanced by online tools and which also augments the teaching role of the librarian.

The many new online products available presented a challenge for health professionals in understanding not only the scope and content of these databases but also basic search competencies. Libraries were challenged to monitor these products, heighten the awareness of health professionals about distinguishing features, and play a role in helping users master the necessary searching skills.

The third-generation OPACs improved functionality dramatically. In a stable environment, activities tend to be grouped by common function within fixed, hierarchical structures, as witnessed in the modular development of bibliographic databases, online catalogs, and information delivery systems. In a rapidly changing environment, one must focus more consciously on the synthesis and integration of these components with specific functions that may not be as easily grouped into distinct categories. In the 1990s, an increasing number of consortia packaged bibliographic databases and document delivery options within the OPAC contract. Libraries shared library systems across institutions, among multiple types of libraries, combining the public and private sectors. By collaborating with other libraries, significantly more resources were made available at a relatively small incremental cost. The development of statewide consortia became more prevalent. One early example is the Ohio Library and Information Network (OhioLINK), a consortium of Ohio college and university libraries formed in 1992 [39].

The reengineered OPAC provided Web access and was more than an incremental change from earlier systems. Functions such as electronic reserves, user-initiated document delivery, user ability to view personal check out records, and the inclusion of tables of contents for books increased the value of the OPAC. It no longer functioned as a self-standing entity but became a gateway to integrated electronic and traditional library resources. By expanding collection development activities, librarians assumed responsibility for a greater diversity of information resources. They assumed new responsibilities, such as assessing the credibility of electronic information available via the Internet, ensuring the currency of information, and identifying and linking to new Web resources. Some libraries offered electronic tables of contents for a high percentage of their books.

The volatility of electronic resources proved to be a major issue during in the late 1990s. Libraries purchased online resources individually and as part of consortia. They received online copies of print resources as part of their print subscriptions. They provided their users access to Web resources. Licensing issues complicated efforts to meet the institution's needs. Measurement and growth of electronic collections continued to be a management problem.

The twenty-first edition of the *Annual Statistics of Medical School Libraries in the United States and Canada*, issued in early 1999, attempts to distinguish print and nonprint serials from their electronic counterparts. The data show the continuing decline of the print format in library collections as well as the ascendancy of the electronic format. In one year, the mean number of reported electronic serials increased over 200%, while the number of unique electronic serials titles increased by 46% over the previous year. Also noteworthy is the number of duplicate serials in light of escalating serial prices. A common practice in the early and mid-1990s was the elimination of duplicate print subscriptions in favor of reserving dollars to maintain the subscription base or to afford new titles. By 1998, however, the trend seemed to reverse, with many health sciences libraries holding duplicate print and electronic subscriptions. The data also reveal the effort by library staff to share the cost of electronic serials. While the number of unique and duplicate electronic titles rose 250% over the previous year, health sciences libraries still held most materials in print format. Much effort and time will be required to make all library resources electronically accessible to users.

As the 1990s unfolded, library homepages on the Web provided a central location for users to locate considerable information on library services in a familiar format. The Web allowed users to obtain information such as self-guided library tours with photographs and hypertext links, library computer-based instruction, guides to using library resources, exhibit materials, online forms to register for classes and request materials, and external pointers to additional Web pages worldwide. This convergence of local resources through the Web enabled users to access many information sources without using multiple software applications and interfaces.

Libraries progressed in their work toward the interoperability of information retrieval systems and the goal of developing robust linkages that are self-healing, redundant, and scalable. As the Internet connected users to a wealth of external public information, comparable needs emerged to connect members of internal communities to restricted information. The institutional intranet addressed these needs and became a more sophisticated replacement for the limited campuswide information systems of the 1980s. Intranets provide access to email and to information or resources placed on a private backbone for the collective group or enterprise.

Libraries were extending both print and electronic collections to larger populations in consortia with the proviso that it not jeopardize service to primary users. As managed care changed the relationship of teaching hospitals, and as the sale of hospitals increased the number of affiliated health professionals in distributed locations, new issues became evident. Three issues critical to health professionals in distributed locations and to health information professionals providing service included user authentication, confidentiality, and information integrity. *Authentication* provides verification that a user has legitimate rights to licensed, published, or private information and that individuals are who they claim to be. *Confidentiality* addresses privacy rights for patients and users of information. Significant clinical and research decisions require *information integrity,* or accuracy and reliability for making decisions that have important outcomes.

The interrelationship of these issues complicated access management for networked information resources. For example, the creation of electronic barricades or firewalls around data may keep select information inside the organization but also prevents the receipt of electronic information from external sources. Administrators face difficult choices to allow legitimate users access to licensed resources and information necessary to perform their jobs. Significant discussions on these issues are taking place among health information professionals [40].

In the 1990s, the increasing availability of networked information resources also triggered a growing interest in the development of distance learning and telemedicine programs. Technologies associated with distance learning remained expensive and attached new significance to questions of who needed to be connected to library resources and how these resources should be made available. Distance learning technology took many forms, such as compressed video, satellite communication, or Web-based instruction. It included many administrative issues, such as online registration, financial management, technological standards, licensing, quality assurance, liability, and political issues.

Distance learning was accompanied by an equally impressive and lengthy list of academic issues. Accreditation required verification that the education delivered to the students at remote sites was equivalent to that provided on campus. This necessitated that data be collected to demonstrate that the two groups did not differ significantly in outcome measures. Faculty required assistance with educational techniques to maximize the use of technology. Planning and coordination were required for both operational issues and the intellectual content. In many instances, librarians assumed responsibility for copyright clearance and electronic reserves, bibliographic instruction, and convenient access to electronic databases. Although, as of early 1999, the electronic copying and scanning of copyrighted works were unsettled areas of the law, there were various models in place for provision of electronic reserves.

Many health sciences libraries obtained copyright permission through the Copyright Clearance Center's (CCC) Electronic Reserves Service, which limited access to the students and instructor of a class. If faculty used Web-based instruction, the faculty member rather than the library was responsible for compliance. The CCC required that records be kept for four full calendar years.

Distance learning introduced a number of interesting innovations. One endeavor to drive a paradigm shift for higher education was the Western Governors University (WGU) [41]. The WGU sought to offer a competency-based, degree-granting virtual university and was introduced by politicians to address the limitations they perceived in traditional higher education. Two major features distinguished the WGU from other distance learning programs: (1) it provided a central clearinghouse for students to identify many available distance learning programs, and (2) it promised to develop its own credentialing and certification programs. To the credit of the WGU design team, libraries were included in the implementation plan from the beginning, although some detractors criticized the shallow information services initially offered to students.

Paralleling the development of distance learning technology was the appearance of telemedicine with its ability to provide immediate access to expert health consultation for an off-site physician. Related to the spread of telemedicine was the High Performance Computing and Communications Act (HPCCA), which created an interagency program to "speed the development of massively parallel, scalable computing systems, ensure connectivity through telecommunications, promote the creation of parallel computer programs and the education of users in these technologies" [42]. The HPCCA provided the platform for the National Information Infrastructure (NII) and its spin-off, the Health Information Infrastructure (HII).

GROWING INTERDEPENDENCE

The 1990s represent a decade of alliances and collaboration among health information professionals. Advances in technology and software, together with a heightened appreciation of self-directed learning, also fostered interest among busy instructors in the use of computer-based multimedia instruction programs [43]. Computer authoring software made it possible for instructors to work with support personnel to put their content rapidly into templates or create new online classes. Software companies welcomed cooperative relationships with developers and provided easy avenues to use their products. Successful program development by instructors was most of all dependent on creating a unified team. Representatives from the library, computing services, educational development, and media production were required to collaborate, with the function of each support unit carefully defined in relation to the others.

Collaboration with health information professionals external to the institution occurred in the 1990s on a much larger scale than previously. The Association of Research Libraries and the two computing organizations CAUSE and EDUCOM formed the Coalition for Networked Information (CNI) in 1990. CNI brought together the content expertise of librarians with the networking expertise of information technologists. The American Medical Informatics Association (AMIA), founded in 1990 through the merger of three existing health information associations, is an organization dedicated to the development and application of medical informatics in the support of patient care, teaching, research, and health care administration. AMIA promotes the development of Internet-based applications and tools for the medical community, provides educational opportunities, and fosters collaboration among clinicians, researchers, information professionals, and policymakers.

The International Coalition of Library Consortia (ICOLC) first met informally as the Consortium of Consortia in 1997. It continues to be an informal self-organized group, composed of (as of August 1998) seventy-nine library consortia in North America but expanding to include the United Kingdom, Germany, the Netherlands, Australia, and other countries. The coalition serves primarily higher education institutions by facilitating discussion among consortia on issues of common interest. ICOLC keeps participating consortia informed about new electronic information resources, pricing practices of electronic providers and vendors, and other issues of importance to directors and governing boards of consortia.

In late 1998, with the help and initiative of information resources leaders at its member institutions, AAMC organized the Group on Information Resources (GIR) for members to share experiences and build the skills necessary to succeed in a technology rich environment. The constituents were composed of chief information officers, vice presidents and senior technology leaders, health sciences library directors, and medical informatics leaders.

In a treatise on medical informatics, Sitting listed several grand challenges for the 1990s [44]. An earlier section in this chapter discussed the development of a unified controlled vocabulary. Sitting added other challenges for medical informatics, including a completely computer-based patient record, the automatic coding of free text reports (such as patient histories), the human genome project, a complete three-dimensional representation of the human body, and techniques to enable the use of information management technologies at the bedside or research bench. This list suggests the importance of employing broad strategic planning techniques across the organization.

In the early 1990s, due to interest from other types of organizations, the NLM broadened the target audience for its IAIMS planning and implementation program. IAIMS initially focused on academic medical centers and was referred to as the Integrated *Academic* Information Management System, but the acronym was changed to Integrated *Advanced* Information Management System to reflect a broader scope. Its enlarged purpose was to promote institution-wide computer networks that linked related library systems to a variety of individual and institutional databases and information files for patient care, research, education, and administration [45].

Technology raises further concerns as to the role of health information professionals in the archiving of electronic documents and planned access to backfiles. Two groups actively pursuing this were OCLC, through its Electronic Collections Online (ECO) service [46], and JSTOR [47]. In its contractual agreements with publishers, OCLC retained the rights to mount all content at OCLC and created a permanent electronic archive. It included the right to store in perpetuity all journal content delivered to OCLC during the period of the contract and to provide ongoing access to libraries that have subscribed to this content, even if the publisher were later to terminate its agreement with OCLC. The JSTOR (short for "Journal Storage") archival project began with a grant from the Mellon Foundation. JSTOR digitized the complete back runs of selected journals in the humanities and social sciences. As of June 2000, it consisted of a database of the images of over 115 journal titles and all but the last three to five years available to subscribers via the Internet.

In spring 2000, yet another electronic archive, named Pub Med Central, emerged as a concept. Pub Med Central is a Web-based repository for barrier-free access to primary reports in the life sciences. It will archive, organize, and distribute peer-reviewed reports from journals, as well as reports that have been screened but not formally peer reviewed. It will coordinate with similar efforts to establish servers internationally, including those overseen by the European Molecular Biology Organization (EMBO). Scientific publishers, professional societies, and other groups independent of the NIH will have complete responsibility for the input to Pub Med Central. Copyright will reside with the submitting groups (i.e., the publishers societies or editorial boards) or the authors themselves, as determined by the participants. Pub Med Central has an advisory committee and selection criteria to ensure submissions of quality.

ROLES, RESPONSIBILITIES, AND RELATIONSHIPS

It is clear that very real changes are occurring within academic and hospital libraries as a result of the impact of technology. However, groups from two schools of thought offer contrasting perspectives on the effect of this technology on the roles, responsibilities, and relationships in which librarians engage. The first group can be referred to as *continuants*. They perceive the changes libraries encounter as "more of the same." The second group will be referred to as *transformationalists*. They perceive recent changes in libraries as truly revolutionary and believe that these changes will alter the world in many ways. In their view, technology coupled with innovation brings about transformation.

As described earlier, librarians are assuming new roles and responsibilities. Are these new roles and responsibilities simply extensions of services that have always been provided? Or is the library's role in the health sciences arena undergoing fundamental metamorphosis? While technology does not function as an independent variable and does not drive changes in isolation, technology is certainly not neutral. In the past, the value of the library centered on its resources. Today value centers on staff abilities, in which the technological knowledge base and required skills continually change. It is therefore essential that libraries support this knowledge base and update staff skills, try new products and services, and monitor developing standards. To meet the challenges of a fluid environment, librarians must be able to recognize and seize nontraditional opportunities for expanded roles. Librarians need not predict what the future will be but rather imagine what they would like it to be [48].

Many library administrators manage computing labs and oversee related areas, such as academic computing and biomedical communication centers. However, roles and responsibilities are changing for those librarians who hold traditional positions as well, such as the enhancement of teaching roles. Librarians not only cope with copyright and licensing of electronic resources but also serve as consultants on these topics for their larger organizations. They not only face the responsibility of shifting from information manager to knowledge manager but must integrate the traditional with the digital library. In particular, hospital librarians serve as experts in health services research. They develop databases of consumer health. They support distance learning and telemedicine. They have become partners on medical informatics research teams and use evidence-based medicine and statistical tools. They serve on appropriate committees within their organizations and within the GIR, AMIA, and CNI.

Librarians develop courses on searching techniques, the use of bibliographic and electronic resources, and finding specialized information on the Internet. Some librarians initiate courses across disciplines. Libraries provide seamless access to resources and databases to support telemedicine efforts, distance learning programs, and users in distributed locations. Librarians develop Web-based modules on bibliographic searching, implement electronic reserves for course materials, and provide materials electronically. Libraries on campuses with distance learning programs demonstrate to accreditation teams that students engaged in remote instruction receive comparable training and resources to those who learn on site. Librarians support telemedicine by increasing physicians' awareness of changing bibliographic tools and consumer health resources that support patient care.

Until 1998, NLM did not consider consumer health within its purview. Health sciences librarians in both academic and hospital settings responded positively to NLM's new emphasis on preventive and consumer health information. Online libraries of health information are emerging to provide the consumer with digitized print materials, access to databases, and online health experts. Netwellness, developed by the University of Cincinnati Medical Center in collaboration with several other partners, reaches a very large population of consumers [49].

Likewise, the role of the health information professional as consultant is expanding with new responsibilities for the development of electronic publications. These products range from electronic newsletters to full, peer-reviewed digital journals without print counterparts. The organization of electronic journals draws on librarians' existing strengths and provides new growth opportunities. Health information professionals provide increased consultation not just on sources of information but on copyright and electronic licensing agreements as well. The steadily increasing number of electronic resources necessitates expertise in appraising licenses to ensure the licensee's rights are protected and an institution's needs are met. Butter points out that librarians need to be aware of the distinction between copyright and contract law and to know who within the institution has the legal authority to sign a contract [50].

In conjunction with other health information professionals, librarians face the daunting task of developing the digital library of the health sciences. The digital library is network based rather than location based. It is also content based and centers on the customer. It generally consists of information storage, retrieval, preservation, access, and delivery components along with knowledge management. The digital library should not be seen as simply a logical and useful extension of the present-day library with an added layer of scientific computing. It represents an entirely new entity. It may contain a genome database component or an electronic journal component that offers services far beyond those of a traditional library.

Lucier predicts that in the next decade librarians will use technology to blend the digital library and the traditional library, which are now separate entities, into an integral whole [51]. He believes the librarian will be more fully integrated into the scholarly and scientific communication process, resulting in a new role called *knowledge management*. The potential to function as knowledge builders grows as librarians provide information support through participation in research teams that use information based techniques such as meta-analysis.

Meta-analysis is an epidemiological and statistical tool used to combine the results of multiple, independent studies. It has been described as "studying the studies" [52]. In a clinical context, meta-analysis synthesizes the various study conclusions to evaluate therapeutic effectiveness, determine procedural efficacy, or provide a basis for the development of treatment protocols. It uses and redefines librarians' data-gathering and organization skills in the creation of firsthand knowledge through research.

Health care reform has brought about a substantial focus on demonstrating quality through the measurement of health outcomes. Health sciences librarians in both hospital and academic settings can become local experts on sources of information for health services research. This makes them extremely valuable members of the health care team. Nearly all health organizations use continuous quality improvement methods to define particular service or problem areas, create process and outcome variables, and institute workplace changes to monitor the effect of new methods or procedures [53]. Such opportunities and techniques play to the skills of librarians.

The WGU and similar online education networks also afford new opportunities. The digital library will do more than provide electronic resources. The challenge of supporting an asynchronous distributed curriculum should excite librarians. They may assume additional responsibilities as a local center providing information services to learners enrolled in a different institution. Key to the implementation of a virtual university such as WGU will be acceptance of WGU credentials, certificates, or degrees by other institutions. How important will the library be in this acceptance? The realization of the virtual university represents a significant paradigm change that will alter the way we think about education and the knowledge base necessary to foster learning.

Library administrators must remain aware of these and other developing roles for health information professionals. Technology has altered what libraries do and how time is spent. It has enlarged the number and variety of people with whom librarians collaborate and compete. It has influenced the way organizations are structured. It is apparent that our behavior is changing as a consequence of the technology that is impacting libraries. Technology influences the way one speaks, the words one uses, and quite possibly one's thought processes. Ong views the word as the basic unit of information exchange rather than a book or computer screen [54]. He proposes that new writing technologies may change the way people think. While technology does not markedly increase our capacity to absorb information, it offers assistance to health information professionals for coping with the increased amount of information and the accelerated pace of change.

Health sciences librarians have a rich history of maximizing technology and adjusting to changing environments, a reputation for collaboration, and a commitment to professional standards and service. Stress in the health sciences librarian's environment has caused modifications to the specialty education responsible for supplying the knowledge and skills required by the profession [55]. By choosing to alter the way they administer human and fiscal resources in light of changing computing, educational, and communication technologies, librarians have become empowered to tackle the challenges of rapid change and emergent possibilities.

IMPACT OF TECHNOLOGY ON THE HUMAN DIMENSION

Library operations continue to increase in technological complexity and face shortening cycles of product obsolescence without any foreseeable return to stability. The continued transformation of libraries requires significant administrative attention to both users and staff. Rather than diminish the need for human interaction, technology calls for an expanded response. Although Chapter 3 of this volume covers the general administration of human resources, no discussion of the impact of technology can overlook five responses the library manager must make in the effective use of automation.

Focusing on the Customer

As technology develops, so do users' expectations. The continued transformation of libraries requires commitment to creating a customer-focused organization. Librarians have traditionally prided themselves on treating users with respect and dignity. However, being customer driven in a technologically changing environment requires more emphasis on responsiveness to the user. Effective librarians recognize what is important to the larger organization, know their users and how the users benefit from their services, and determine the services that truly add value. These librarians actively solicit feedback from users and devise new responses to the changing institutional milieu.

Measuring Performance

Seymour points out that "feedback without measurement is just opinion; measurement without feedback is just data" [56]. Both are needed. Recognizing that the provision of input and output measures are no longer enough in the managed care arena, today's librarians grapple with defining meaningful outcome measures. As imperfect as survey, focus groups, and other methods of measurement may be, they yield useful insights. Complemented with anecdotal evidence, these measures enable librarians to assess current practice and determine whether the right service is being provided.

Librarians also learn from the experiences of others. The Association of Academic Health Sciences Libraries has collected data on an annual basis since fiscal year 1974/75. Libraries have traditionally used these statistics to compare themselves with the libraries of peer institutions, but these statistics also may serve as a point of departure for establishing benchmarks and determining criteria for performance measures for the academic health sciences library. For example, librarians could examine ILL efforts, such as the fill rate, the cost of providing service, and turnaround time for delivery. It may be found that libraries with the best services have certain attributes, such as intensive use of technology, or have redesigned every process. From this analysis, one could determine an appropriate benchmark and redesign ILL services accordingly.

Another example of focusing on performance measures would be the use of pre- and posttests in educational sessions with subsequent follow-up. Counting the number of individuals attending classes is an indirect measure of benefit, but surveying attendees three months after the class measures what content was actually retained and used. Identifying best practices through the literature and through professional contacts enables the benchmarking of training and services against other national groups.

Realigning the Organization

Technology has impacted organizations on a much larger scale than may be immediately apparent. The traditional concepts of span of control and hierarchical reporting are predicated on the belief that communication cannot be rich and broad simultaneously. Jobs in industry, health care, and libraries have been structured to channel large amounts of customized information to a few people in the hierarchy, with much less information going to the larger group of employees. Technologically improved communications broaden the base of people who can receive this rich communication. Evans and Wurster discuss how these changes occur at differing rates and with varying intensity in industry [57]. Changes in communication have proceeded concurrently with organizational realignments.

Parallels can be seen within libraries. Although "director" continues to be the most common title for the administrator of the library, since 1994 numerous health sciences library directors have incorporated other institutional functions into their sphere of influence. Hospital library directors experienced this expansive trend even earlier. These differing responsibilities for units outside the library are reflected in a wide variety of titles, such as associate vice chancellor for health affairs, director of library and biomedical communications, assistant dean for education research, and assistant dean for information resources. At the same time, individuals with medical degrees, second master's degrees, and doctoral degrees now direct some libraries.

As health information professionals, librarians increasingly work with a wider variety of players (e.g., informaticists, departmental or clinical computing units, and researchers), depending on the needs and priorities of the parent institution. Consequently, it may be fair to say that health sciences libraries, at least for the short run, are becoming more dissimilar. As they become more dissimilar, measuring what libraries do and defining meaningful benchmarks becomes more challenging. This places greater importance on the ability to think critically about the application of technology.

Because technological change is occurring so quickly, administrators must create flexible organizations. This generally translates as fewer layers, fewer rules, and employees empowered to respond to customers [58]. Less hierarchical organization structures are better able to respond to change. Block stresses that administrators must be powerful advocates for their units while not alienating those around or above them [59]. Health information professionals require both the technological skills that convey confidence and the process skills to develop mutual understanding and trust. The health sciences librarian must combine technical skills with leadership and organizational skills.

Creating a Learning Environment

A library administrator cannot resolve all the complexities brought on by rapidly changing technology. Instead, one must provide the training, resources, and a learning environment to instill in the staff a desire to address these issues. All professionals involved in implementing information technology innovations need to be taught contemporary management methods for humanizing the workplace in light of technology [60]. Too many people in all sectors of the workplace feel overwhelmed by the onslaught of unending technological change. Although people can do almost anything for a short period of time, heroic effort is not a sustainable model of operation. Much of the literature addressing the effect of technology on people uses the term *technostress* [61], and the effective administrator will strive to counter it.

Lorenzi and others have noted that "the cornerstone of all interpersonal transactions is treating people with respect through honesty and trust" [62]. From that foundation one can build what Senge refers to as the learning organization, a workplace that requires new ideas and the application of new knowledge to ongoing activities [63]. A learning environment involves staff in the change process. By systematically looking at the possibilities of automated systems, asking questions, and trying to find answers, staff can improve services and work processes.

Businesses have found that people in organizations act collectively but learn individually. Documentation of best practices often leaves out the mistakes that people learn from and obscures the hidden logic and struggles that have made breakthroughs possible [64]. One method for overcoming the conundrum of collective learning is the learning history developed by the Massachusetts Institute of Technology's Center for Organizational Learning. The learning history consists of a written narrative or first-person account that captures a critical event or change [65]. The history can be analyzed and used as a basis for group discussion by those involved in the process as well as those who might learn from it.

Renewing the Knowledge Base

Continuous improvement requires a commitment to learning [66]. Librarians have been long-term advocates of continuing education and lifelong learning. Covey refers to the continuous process of self-renewal as the *inside-out theory* [67]. One must renew one's own knowledge base and nurture a learning work environment. The Medical Library Association has identified skills required by today's librarian and advocated that lifelong learning must be a personal imperative and institutional strategy [68]. Despite the many pressures to perform within libraries and the larger institutional environment, librarians also must remember that they are part of a larger profession and have an obligation to give back. Librarians invest in the future by making a conscious and continuous commitment as mentors, committee members, and contributors to the professional knowledge base.

FINANCIAL IMPLICATIONS OF TECHNOLOGY

Technology impacts all aspects of the library budget. While each successive generation of information technology brings new levels of performance and functionality, overall costs for technology increase. In accepting the exponential growth of technology, library administrators much develop financial and management strategies to accommodate it. The budget remains the most powerful tool to ensure that institutional plans are implemented and contributions are rewarded [69]. By linking the budget to strategic plans within the framework of institutional values, the administrator manages scarce fiscal resources and makes optimal use of technology in both the long and short term.

In recent years, libraries have witnessed major changes in the financing of technology, electronic collections, and personnel costs. The paradigm for managing technology assets has shifted from obtaining large infusions of capital every five to ten years to budgeting more evenly dispersed and smaller amounts on an ongoing basis. Typically, libraries have bought hardware and amortized computer investments over as many years as possible. Now the library may be better served through leasing or buying the smallest computer to do the job with plans to upgrade it.

The economic life cycle of technology may be defined as the useful financial life of an item as determined by its age, the plan to keep it, or the projection as to when the item will no longer be suited for its intended purpose [70]. Life cycles are getting shorter. Projecting the useful life for information technology equipment may not be easy. However, keeping equipment too long raises maintenance costs and forfeits the advantages of new technology. At some point, replacement becomes cheaper than maintenance and support.

In considering replacement, one differentiates between price and cost. The price is what is paid to make a purchase. The cost includes the price as well as other expenses associated with owning, operating, and maintaining the item. A lower cost per unit for individual components of a computer system does not always translate into a lower acquisition price for today's average automated system. While the price per unit of memory, processors, and most peripherals has fallen dramatically, one seldom buys an exact replacement. Instead, libraries frequently buy automated systems that increase the functionality as well as the total cost. The best technology solutions support future cost avoidance rather than cost reduction.

Turning to information content, the pricing of materials in the electronic environment is complex and highly volatile. Despite discussions of imminent trends toward obtaining information based on a transactional model, the many cost advantages of bundling like items together do not go away with electronic journals. Journals represent bundles of articles, and there are good

marketing reasons for publishers to bundle [71]. Although bundling complicates collection development decisions, it has encouraged libraries to license
electronic resources through consortia. When negotiating collective agreements, however, it is most important to know the specific needs of your institution and the bottom line [72].

Technology also impacts the personnel budget. Libraries now hire a
broader spectrum of people, all of whom need to be compensated according to the work performed. In many positions, a greater emphasis must be
placed on skills than degrees. Libraries face new costs for ongoing training,
user support, and time to reconfigure networks. Support for lifelong learning and staff development is needed for all levels of staff. Given that the total
cost of owning technology is rising, administrators need to augment the
budget to support the necessary technology. One strategy is to reallocate
current budgets and emphasize aggressive waste management. Alternatively,
linking costs to funding sources may drive new funding formulas for electronic collections, staff compensation, expensing depreciation, and additional investments in technology.

In some institutions, services considered basic to users may be completely subsidized while optional services may be subsidized at a lower
rate or require complete cost recovery. Some institutions elect to outsource
entire systems to larger institutions that act as a broker for services. Library
operating budgets are impacted by new costs resulting from enhancements
in technology or from another unit's effort to transfer costs. For example,
many library operations budgets have been negatively affected by increased paper costs resulting from the need to print electronic information
stored on servers. This situation has resulted in libraries installing systems
to charge users for the prints they make. Health sciences librarians now
make many organizational decisions about technology cost subsidization
in light of service goals.

LEADING THE PROCESS OF CHANGE

To compete in today's information society, library administrators are required to be visionary and goal oriented. They must educate top management to the opportunities that information technology offers the organization, as well as the strategic issues that must be addressed. Libraries must
demonstrate value. They must ensure quality outcomes within institutions
and the larger health care arena by managing knowledge at the earliest
phases of the research process and by connecting people to information they
would not otherwise have. Lifelong learning skills must be taught. Through
these efforts, libraries save users time, a most precious commodity in the
health sciences environment.

Administrators must be politically adept in acquiring resources without alienating peers, administrators, or users. They must remain current on technology issues, open to change, and be prepared to embrace new opportunities. Because of change, past methods may no longer work. Successful leaders will distinguish which activities require a fundamental rethinking and will deliver dramatic improvement. Interpersonal skills and the ability to negotiate carry equal importance. Librarians need to create new electronic information resources, establish new information delivery platforms, and work with new players. They need to be creative and curious in testing new resources.

Assumptions cannot go unchallenged. Librarians must continue to participate in the development of and adherence to professional standards. Administrators must be sensitive to the impact technology and associated changes have on staff, compensate appropriately, and provide support to maintain expertise to thrive with changing roles. Health information professionals must remain advocates of lifelong learning and other values of the profession. Practicing evidence-based librarianship can improve the direct outcome of services.

Technology enhances the ability to connect people with information and enables libraries to increase the emphasis on evaluating services. With the assistance of technology, librarians can withstand scrutiny and become agents of change not only within but also throughout their institutions. The challenges posed by technology are great, but so are the opportunities to truly make a difference within the larger environment. Health information professionals are limited only by their imagination. Never before has technology provided such powerful tools, and health sciences librarians can create a rewarding future despite the rapidity of change.

REFERENCES

1. Braude RM. On the origin of a species: evolution of health sciences librarianship. Bull Med Libr Assoc 1997 Jan;85(1):1-10.

2. Matheson NW. The idea of the library in the twenty-first century. Bull Med Libr Assoc 1995 Jan;83(1):1-7.

3. Anderson RK. Rachael Keller Anderson, Medical Library Association president 1997-98. Bull Med Libr Assoc 1998 Apr;86(2):293-4.

4. Braude RM. Personal communication, March 17, 2000.

5. Peay WJ. Strategies and measures for our next century. Bull Med Libr Assoc 1999 Jan;87(1):1-8.

6. Medical Library Association. Code of Ethics for Health Sciences Librarianship. [Web document]. Chicago: Medical Library Association, 1996. Available from Internet: http://www.mlanet.org/about/ethics.html.

7. Brodman E. Pragmatism and intellection in medical library education. In: Berk RA, ed. Proceedings of the Allerton Invitational Conference on Education for Health

Sciences Librarianship, April 2-4, 1979, Monticello, Illinois. Chicago: Medical Library Association, 1979:viii-xv.

8. Tapscott D, Caston A. Paradigm shift: the new promise of information technology. New York: McGraw-Hill, 1993.

9. Pizer, I. Looking backward, 1984-1959: Twenty-five years of library automation, a personal view. Bull Med Libr Assoc 1984 Oct;72(4):335-48.

10. Bunting A. From Index Catalogue to Gopher space: changes in our profession as reflected in the Handbook and CPHSL. Bull Med Libr Assoc 1994 Jan;82(21):1-11.

11. Rutkowski AM. Internet. Seattle, WA: Microsoft® Encarta® 98 Encyclopedia, 1998.

12. Ibid., 4.

13. National Library of Medicine. Fact Sheets. [Web document]. Available from Internet: http://www.ncbi.nlm.nih.gov/pubmed.

14. Brodman E, Johnson MF Jr. Medical serials control systems by computer: a state of the art review. Bull Med Libr Assoc 1976 Jan;64(1):12-19.

15. Pizer, op. cit., 340.

16. Gurwitt R. Council on Library Resources, Inc.: 37th Annual Report. Special insert. Washington, DC: Council on Library Resources, 1993:7.

17. University of California, Berkeley. Computing Services. The MELVYL online library catalog. Berkeley: University of California Press, 1985.

18. Kelly E, Fedders C, Powderly A, Yedlin D. Bibliographic access and control system. Inf Tech Libr 1982 Jun;1(2):125-32.

19. Broering NC. The Georgetown University library information system (LIS): a minicomputer based integrated library system. Bull Med Libr Assoc 1983 Jul;71(3):317-23.

20. Blois MS, Shortliffe EH. The computer meets medicine: emergence of a discipline. In: Shortliffe EH, Pereault LE, Widerhold G, and Fagan L, eds. Medical informatics: computer applications in health care. Reading, MA: Addison-Wesley, 1990:3-36.

21. Warner HR. Medical informatics: a real discipline? J Am Med Inform Assoc 1995 Jul/Aug;2(4): 207-8.

22. Johnson MF Jr., Pride RB. OCTANET: an electronic library network. I. Design and development. Bull Med Libr Assoc 1983 Apr;71(2):184-91.

23. Crawford S, Johnson MF Jr., Kelly EA. Technology at Washington University School of Medicine Library: BACS, PHILSOM, and OCTANET. Bull Med Libr Assoc 1983 Jul;71(3):324-7.

24. Miller J. How are libraries using QuickDoc? Results of a national survey of QuickDocUsers. J Int Loan Doc Del Info Supply1995; 5(3):71-88.

25. Woodsmall RM, Lyon-Hartmann B, Siegel ER, eds. MEDLINE on CD-ROM: National Library of Medicine evaluation forum, Bethesda, Maryland, September 2, 1988. Medford, NJ: Learned Information, 1989.

26. Physicians for the twenty-first century: report of Project Panel on the General Professional Education of the Physician and College Preparation for Medicine. J Med Educ 1984 Nov;59(2):1-208.

27. Florance V, Braude RM, Frisse ME, Fuller S. Educating physicians to use the digital library. Acad Med 1995 Jul;71(7): 597-602.

28. Frisse ME. Medical informatics in academic health science centers. Acad Med 1992 Apr;67(4):238-41.

29. Fuller S, Braude RM, Florance V, Frisse M. Managing information in the academic medical center: building an integrated information environment. Acad Med 1995 Oct;70(10): 887-91.

30. Frisse ME, Braude RM, Florance V, Fuller S. Informatics and medical libraries: changing needs and changing roles. Acad Med 1995 Jan;70(1):30-5.

31. Selden, CR, Humphries BL. Unified Medical Language System (UMLS). [Web document]. Available from Internet: http://www.nlm.nih.gov/research/umls/umls-main.html.

32. Association of Academic Health Sciences Library Directors. Committee on Library Information Management Technology. Report on automation activities of member libraries. [Seattle, WA: Association of Academic Health Sciences Library Directors, 1987].

33. Rutkowski, op. cit., 4.

34. Schoch NA. Communication on a listserv for health information professionals: uses and users of MEDLIB-L. Bull Med Libr Assoc 1997;85(1):23-32.

35. Landes S. The ARIEL document delivery system: a cost-effective alternative to the fax J Int Loan Doc Del Info Supply 1997;7(3):61-72.

36. Basch, R. Uncover. Link-Up. 1995 Nov/Dec;12(6):12-13.

37. Association of American Medical Colleges. Medical school objectives project: medical informatics objectives. [Web document]. Available from Internet: http://www.aamc.org/meded/msop/informat.htm.

38. Sackett D, Richardson WS, Rosenberg W, et al. Evidence-based medicine: how to practice and teach EBM. New York: Harcourt, Brace: 1998:5.

39. Cook A, Barber D. Ohio Library and Information Network: OhioLINK. [Web document]. Available from Internet: http://www.ohiolink.edu/.

40. Lynch C. Access management for networked information resources. 1998. [Web document]. Available from Internet: http://www.arl.org/newsltr/201/cni.html.

41. Peay, op cit., 2.

42. Lindberg DA, Humphreys BL. Computers in medicine. JAMA 1995 Jun 7;273(21):1667-8.

43. Hart JK. Self-directed learning program and the library: supporting instructors in development of multimedia instructional programs. Bull Med Libr Assoc 1994 Oct;82(4):434.

44. Sitting, D. Grand challenges in medical informatics. J Am Med Inform Assoc 1995 Jul/Aug;1(5):412-3.

45. National Library of Medicine. Fact sheets. [Web document]. Available from Internet: http://www.nlm.nih.gov/pubs/factsheets/iaims.html.

46. Archiving ensures perpetual access to electronic collections online. OCLC Newsletter 1997 Jul/Aug;228:28.

47. Guthrie KM, Lougee WP. The JSTOR solution: accessing and preserving the past. Lib J 1997 Feb 1;122:42-4.

48. Dougherty RM, Hughes C. Preferred futures for libraries: a summary of six workshops with university provosts and library directors. Berkeley, CA: Research Libraries Group, Inc., 1991.

49. Guard R, Haag D, Kaya B, Marine S, et al. An electronic consumer health library: NetWellness. Bull Med Libr Assoc 1996 Oct;84(4):468-77.

50. Butter, K. Electronic licensing: a presentation at the Medical Library Association meeting. May 1997.

51. Lucier RE. Knowledge management: redefining the roles in scientific communication. EDUCOM Rev 1990 Fall;25(3):21-7.

52. Mead TL, Richards DT. Librarian participation in meta-analysis projects. Bull Med Libr Assoc 1995 Oct;83(4):461-4.

53. Masys DR. The informatics of health care reform. Bull Med Libr Assoc 1996 Jan;84(1):11-6.

54. Ong, WJ. Writing is a technology that restructures thought. In: Baumann G, ed. The written word: literacy in transition. Oxford: Oxford University Press, 1986:23-50.

55. Braude, op cit., 2.

56. Seymour D. Once upon a campus: lessons for improving quality and productivity in higher education. Phoenix: American Council on Education/Oryx Press, 1995.

57. Evans PB, Wurster TS. Strategy and the new economics of information. Harv Bus Rev 1997 Sep-Oct;75(5):71-82.

58. Ibid., 74.

59. Block P. The empowered manager: positive political skills as work. San Francisco: Jossey-Bass, 1987.

60. Ash J. Organizational factors that influence information technology diffusion in academic health sciences centers. J Am Med. Inform Assoc 1997 Mar-Apr;4(2):108.

61. Osif BA, Harwood RA. Technostress. Lib Adm Manage 1996;10(1):44-7.

62. Lorenzi NM, Riley RT, Blyth AJ, Southon G, et al. Antecedents of the people and organizational aspects of medical informatics: review of the literature. J Am Med Inform Assoc 1997 Mar/Apr;4(2):88.

63. Senge PM. The fifth discipline: the art and practice of the learning organization. New York: Doubleday/Currency, 1990.

64. Kleiner A, Roth G. How to make experience your company's best teacher. Harv Bus Rev1997 Sep-Oct;75(5):172-7.

65. Ibid., 174-5.

66. Garvin, DA. Building a learning organization. Harv Bus Rev 1993 Jul-Aug;71:78-91.

67. Covey SR. First things first. New York: Simon and Schuster, 1994.

68. Platform for change: the educational policy statement of the Medical Library Association. Chicago: Medical Library Association, 1991.

69. Association of Governing Boards of Universities and Colleges. The time for strategic budgeting has come. NCHEMS News 1995 Oct:12.

70. Oberlin JL. Financial mythology of information technology: the new economics. Cause/Effect 1996 Spring;19(1):22-9.

71. Varian HR. Pricing Information goods. 1995 Jun. [Web document]. Available from Internet: http://www.sims.berkeley.edu/resources/infoecon.

72. Fisher R, Ury W. Getting to yes: negotiating agreement without giving in. Boston: Houghton Mifflin, 1991.

6

Planning for Health Sciences Library Facilities

Frieda O. Weise and Mary Joan (M.J.) Tooey

Health sciences libraries today sit at a pivotal point in their history and development. Therefore, the task of planning a new facility for the twenty-first century demands vision and leadership, flexibility, and resourcefulness. It presents challenging and satisfying responsibilities for a librarian, and it certainly can be a career highlight. Developments in information and communications technologies already have had a profound effect on library functions and services, challenging the very idea of a library. The uncertainly as to the degree to which electronic information will overtake or replace print information makes one wish for a crystal ball. Jesse Shera said that the objective of the library is to bring together human beings and recorded knowledge in as fruitful a relationship as humanly possible [1]. This remains a valid objective in the era of electronic information.

In this chapter we seek to provide practical guidance to librarians planning a new health sciences library. Many of these tenets apply equally to a renovation or addition. The suggested readings contain numerous references to renovation. The chapter will highlight issues of paramount importance in planning health sciences library space that will endure into the twenty-first century. Discussion will cover the essential steps in the planning process, from writing the program plan to moving into the new facility. Although some librarians will have the good fortune to be involved in all these steps, the chapter is organized so that the reader can focus on the details most relevant to a given situation. A selected list of suggested readings contains planning principles and guidelines as well as more specific problems, such as interior design and planning for technology. This chapter does not repeat the sound information in classic works such as Metcalf [2] or the carefully written chapter by Hitt [3] in the fourth edition of the *Handbook of Medical Library Practice.*

Our direct experience has shaped the content of this chapter. Having recently been involved in planning a new health sciences library/information center that integrates library and computing services, we have experience in both the practical and political aspects of such a venture. Working with others will be reiterated as an essential strategy in all steps of a building project. Regardless of the institutional setting, rarely will the librarian be totally responsible for the planning process. It is important to include as many staff, consultants, and others as possible; to listen or read to learn from others' mistakes; to seek advice and guidance; and to stand firm when you think you are right based on the evidence.

GENERAL CONSIDERATIONS

Planning a health sciences library facility that will function effectively in the twenty-first century requires careful examination of the mission of the library and how it is likely to change over the next several decades. For example, libraries have traditionally been designed to provide enough space for twenty years of growth of a print collection. This premise may no longer be valid in the face of electronic resources and alternative ways of storing and retrieving scholarly information.

Before any actual planning begins, we strongly recommend allocating time to bring together institutional administrators with librarians to discuss issues that have architectural implications. This provides an opportunity to educate administrators on the importance of connectivity, service points, electronic resources, the continuing need for print material, and other issues. Philosophical considerations about the function and purpose of the library affect the architecture of the facility. The library may well reflect the vision and aspirations of the institution. It may be the landmark or signature building that is the focal point of the campus or a marketing point for other health care settings.

Libraries provide access to information and services through information and communications technologies systems. The infrastructure design must be flexible enough to incorporate future technological needs while addressing current specific functions. For example, user areas featuring multimedia stations may replace stacks later. Plans should allow for flexibility in wiring, lighting, and functions over time. As library users employ information technologies traditionally provided by computer centers, thought should be given to the possible merging of these functions in one facility. Libraries can address the need for one-stop information shopping by providing the information, the technology, and the instruction in its use all in one location. Students still will need a well-designed facility for study, both individually and in groups. The current trend in problem-based learning in health sciences professional education places a great demand on libraries for group study space. Students with laptops require access to power and data connections. Furthermore, local developments in distance education should be considered, because libraries are an ideal location to provide this type of learning environment and, with the appropriate technology, can be the gateway to and from remote sites.

Finally, print publications can be expected to remain with us for the next generation of health sciences libraries buildings. Electronic journal publication and distribution are at an early phase of evolution, and retrospective conversion of all existing print collections is not likely. Consequently, libraries will need to house print collections for the near future. A recent trend has been to provide access to materials, rather than owning them. To be sure, access through interlibrary loan, commercial document delivery services, or full-text electronic journals is a factor in facility planning and depends on budgets and expenses as well as the needs of faculty and students. Remote storage for older collections can also be considered to reduce the amount of stack space required.

Mark Twain wrote, "The reports of my death are greatly exaggerated," when reading a premature obituary [4]. The talk about the death of libraries is greatly exaggerated as well. The "virtual" library is not yet a practical reality. A library facility plan must include a blend of space for public access and use, staff, technology, and print collections.

PREPARING FOR PLANNING

Many types of planning occur while building a new library facility or renovating an existing one. Such a project requires planning for the building, fund-raising, moving staff and materials, and many other aspects. In the following discussion, *planning* will refer to the planning process leading up to the actual construction of the building. This process encompasses the preparatory phase of writing the building program plan, selection of the architects, program verification, and schematic and design development. Additionally, changes in the design can take place throughout the construction process, contingent on the budget and the patience of everyone involved. Planning of a more pragmatic nature continues during the construction phase as final decisions unfold concerning furnishings, interior design, and the movement and final placement of collections, staff, and services. These planning concerns are addressed later in the chapter.

THE BUILDING PROGRAM PLAN

Writing the program plan may take place years before the actual selection of architects or construction of the building. In some cases, the program plan is amended over the years; in others, it is continuously rewritten. In some cases, the program plan may be written as part of the base architectural services upon startup of the project.

The building program plan puts forth a vision for the building and sets the direction for attaining that vision. According to Metcalf, the building program is "the comprehensive document describing and detailing the library building and its space requirements, its philosophy of service, functional areas and relationships, and spatial content and details as needed to communicate to the architects the desires of the owner-user" [5]. Requirements for a formal program plan vary from institution to institution. The program plan may be a very formal document mandated by the parent organization or funding agency, or it may consist of a few pages stating why a new facility is needed. Whether or not a formal program is required, it behooves a library director to write down thoughts concerning the facility's needs, if only to clarify the issues in her mind. A well-thought-out, articulate, organized, and prepared document can ensure the success of the project. It can be used to secure funding and serve as a guidepost for development of the project through all phases. The owner and architect use this document to develop a common understanding of the goals and language of the project.

Writing the Program Plan

Because the program plan carries such importance, the prospect of writing it may appear daunting. In many institutions, facilities management or institutional planning units exist to provide direction or dictate a template or formula for the document. In some cases, these units actually write the program plan. However, the need for involvement and continuous input from the library director and staff cannot be overemphasized. Staff need to assist in the planning and have continuous input into the project; involving all levels of staff in its preparation also builds a feeling of understanding and ownership in the program.

During the writing process, it can be useful to hire a library consultant. Although it is essential to have a consultant during later planning stages, hiring one to assist in the preparation of the program plan often is overlooked or is omitted as a cost-saving measure. A library consultant can review the document upon its completion to ensure the inclusion of important elements. In many institutions, the program plan can be received as "written in stone" with little deviation allowed from the completed document. A consultant or, at the very least, another experienced, impartial colleague, may save steps later.

Building program elements vary from institution to institution. Common elements include

- a description of the project;
- the need for and expected contribution to institutional services, including

a general description of the current facility and its inadequacies, and the current needs for collection, users, and services, staff, and technology;
- general building considerations, including the site;
- spatial relationships, such as departments that need to be adjacent to core elements (e.g., elevators, mail rooms, or loading docks);
- descriptions of individual areas, such as cataloging, reference, public computing; and
- appendices containing useful information about the library such as staff size, workloads, and projections for five, ten, or twenty years [6].

This program plan structure affords an opportunity to address philosophical issues in libraries and also to present statistics reflecting growth in collections, services, and user populations to assist in building the case for a new or renovated facility. It represents a critical opportunity to articulate actual needs in terms of staff, collection, and user spaces. It necessitates time and thought, the ability to project into the future, and prediction of the spatial and programmatic needs of a building that may be built for a thirty-year life span.

Fortunately, numerous resources aid in this process. Titles in Appendix B, Annotated Bibliography of Library Space Planning, contain examples from program plans. In addition to monographs, the journal literature provides current, helpful discussions concerning directions for technology and its impact on space and services. The computing, communications, and education literature gives useful trend information concerning the use of technology. Additionally, annual features in the *Bulletin of the Medical Library Association, Library Journal,* and *American Libraries* focus on new construction. The Library Administration and Management Association (LAMA) of ALA has a Web site devoted to the topic: www.ala.org/LAMA/publications/list. Information from colleagues who have planned new buildings or renovations can be invaluable. Some share their program plan. Finally, visiting new or renovated facilities adds invaluable, multifaceted information. A visit may uncover programmatic elements that were overlooked. Design elements such as office layout and decor, colors, seating, and window coverings should be noted and stored for reference during later stages of the project.

FUNDING NEEDS

Building budgets differ from institution to institution, however, elements common to all projects include the following:

- Preconstruction funds or planning monies, which are used for program verification, schematic design, and design development
- Construction funds, which provide funding for the actual building of the facility and may include demolition of existing structures or site preparation

- Funding for equipment and furnishings such as furniture and shelving, which may not cover high-technology items or photocopiers, depending on restrictions of the governing agency; for example, in Maryland, the category of capital equipment does not include anything with less than a fifteen-year life span or anything that is mobile
- Consultants' fees; although many architectural firms hire a consultant, the library should retain a consultant of its own to ensure objective advice from an experienced, knowledgeable person
- Moving and relocation costs that may not appear in the funding allocated for the construction of a new facility and may need to come out of the library's operating budget; it is good to know the allocation of these costs early so that extra funding may be requested
- Miscellaneous items, such as architectural renderings, models, brochures, slides, and special events such as the library opening

FUNDING SOURCES

The funding for a facility may or may not be an issue and will come from various sources, depending on the institution. In a state-affiliated institution, funding may have to be approved by a governmental source such as the state legislature or board of public works. This funding allotment may be tied to a formula based on square footage with little room for negotiation. The actual monies may come from the state construction funding, bonds, gifts, or a combination of sources. Likewise, in a private institution financing may come from institutional general funds or donors. In either setting, it may be necessary to participate in fund-raising activities. If construction monies are limited, it may become necessary to raise funds for furnishings, equipment, or special spaces.

Some of the steps in the fund-raising process include building fund-raising boards, developing campaign timelines, writing case statements, planning special events, and developing campaign materials. Another time-consuming aspect involves visits by, and presentations to, potential donors. If possible, identify funding and naming opportunities in a variety of price ranges. Although it is advantageous to have donations for concrete items, the development of unrestricted endowments also is attractive in an era of rapid technological change. Lee [7] and Steele [8] have written useful books, and Chapter 2, Fiscal Management in Health Sciences Libraries, includes a general discussion of fund-raising.

THE SITE

In an ideal world, every library would be centrally located on the campus or within the institution and equally accessible to every user. It would have ample, free, and close parking for all constituents, and it would be safe and secure. The site would not place any limitations on the shape or height of the building. However, the real world poses many restrictions. In urban areas land is often at a premium and expensive. Where land is available, it may not be in the center of the campus and may be located far from some user groups. A project within an existing building, such as a new or renovated hospital library, may face severe restrictions on the amount of available space. Other departments may compete fiercely for the square footage.

For example, the new Health Sciences and Human Services Library at the University of Maryland, Baltimore Campus (UMBC), faced several site restrictions. Because of its location in an urban area, land for a new facility was hard to obtain and had a number of drawbacks. It was not centrally located and was shaped like an elongated rectangle, necessitating a long and narrow building, which is not the most efficient for the provision of services. The site also had a height restriction because of the flight path for MEDEVAC helicopters. On the positive side, the site was close to parking and highly visible to visitors to Baltimore, thus affording the opportunity to design a high-profile, signature building for the campus.

STEPS IN THE PROJECT PLANNING PROCESS

The planning process encompasses many components, from composing a planning team to choosing an architect; negotiating fees; identifying collection, public, and staff and service space needs; and determining document delivery and resources management strategies. These and several additional topics are discussed in the following sections.

The Planning Team

The planning team will ultimately be responsible for creating an aesthetically pleasing and functional building. In other words, the library should be effective both internally and externally. As Metcalf points out, tastes and circumstances change, but a good building can serve the needs of the institution over a long period of time [9].

The planning team can be composed of many groups and individuals, representing different interests and bringing different knowledge and skills to the process. It is likely that the whole team will rarely meet at the same time but must be coordinated over months or even years to reach its goal. The planning process may become highly political, depending on the stakeholders, all of whom wish the building to reflect well on them. It is extremely important to establish and maintained rapport among library planners, architects, institutional planners, and other working committees. All participants must respect each other's perspectives and be able to compromise. The role of the planning team should be fully understood by all participants.

Several good discussions regarding the planning team can be found in Metcalf [10], Hitt [11], and Somerville [12]. Metcalf provides an excellent overview of the many types of committees, while Somerville describes the planning process in some detail. Hitt provides a succinct overview of some of the key players. The following discussion describes the most likely groups and individuals who should participate on the planning team and their roles.

Library Planners

Responsibility for coordinating the library's role in the planning process should be assigned to a specific person. Depending on the setting, this could be the library director or another person from the library staff designated as the project manager. It cannot be overemphasized that one person should coordinate discussion among all the planning groups and represent the library's interest in an assertive but tactful manner. The project manager must be readily available because demands frequently are deadline driven and urgent. This consumes large amounts of an individual's time, and the assignment should take this into consideration. The project manager serves as the focal point for communication and contact with the architects, consultants, library staff, interior designers, the institution's facility planners, and advisory committees. If the person is not the director, the manager needs to communicate all activities to the director and reflect to others the director's wishes.

Library Staff

Members of the library staff must be actively involved in the planning process. The library may choose to have a representative committee, but it is important that all staff have an opportunity to participate and give input in some form because

- they are knowledgeable about how users access services;
- they understand internal library functions and how their offices and work areas operate for maximum efficiency;
- they will spend their working life in the building;
- they are well versed in library trends, new roles, technologies, and how users and functions may be affected; and
- they can contribute insights and solutions to potential design problems [13].

Architects

The architects may be the last group to join the planning team because in many institutions significant planning or programming takes place prior to their selection. It is important that the architects and library planners develop a positive relationship early in the process so that library functions can be reviewed in detail. Many architects are not familiar with library functions, and several meetings may be necessary to discuss functions, spatial relationships, and other functions. A good working relationship facilitates negotiation and compromise during the design and construction stages. It is imperative that the architects be advised of the site and space constraints and how the building will fit into the institution's master facilities plan as they begin to develop the aesthetic design. Selection of the architects will be discussed further in a later section.

Consultants

Because a library building is an expensive investment, having an experienced, unbiased outside opinion avoids mistakes. Normally, library staff and other institutional planners do not have experience with planning a building; sometimes the architects have limited experience with libraries. Some of the benefits to hiring a consultant include additional knowledge and expertise; objectivity and analytical skills; provision of influence to help sell the project; time savings for the library staff; assumption of the role of educator, facilitator, or change agent; and the introduction of new ideas and perspectives to foster a creative ferment among the planners. An effective building consultant brings broad, diversified experience to the project and current knowledge of building planning, design, and furnishings. Consultants also need a certain degree of political acumen combined with good group process and interpersonal skills. Because much of the work that a consultant does involves reporting and recording, the consultant should have good documentation, writing, and presentation skills [14]. Normally, the consultant is hired by the organization; however, some architectural firms hire consultants to assist their planners. Hitt points out three important reasons to hire a consultant: (1) he or she can serve as a sounding board for the library's ideas; (2) an outside observer can present objective alternatives that the local planning team can overlook; (3) as an objective third party, the consultant can help settle differences of opinion when controversies arise [15].

In addition to the library building consultant, the architectural firm will most likely retain consultants in interior and landscape design, lighting, computing, and structural, mechanical, and electrical engineering firms. These consultants will be hired for specific stages of the project and also will interact with the planning team. Metcalf offers a thorough discussion of these types of consultants [16].

Other Groups

Depending on the institutional setting, other agencies or groups, such as donors, may be included in planning for political reasons. Donors may require that their funds be used in a specific way and dictate uses for space.

For example, one donor required a leisure reading room in a research library; another a prominent facility for rare books. Donors may also have strong, even bizarre, opinions regarding furnishings or colors. Trustees or state governing agency may mandate review by others. For example, typical of many states, Maryland requires that the Department of General Services and an architectural review board approve all designs. The University of Maryland, Baltimore Campus, also retains an external firm of value engineers to review the plans for possible cost savings.

Internal Planners

1. *Users:* Because the library's ultimate purpose is to meet the needs of its users, their requirements, desires, and use patterns must be understood. Although library staff monitor and try to anticipate user needs, users desire a direct voice in the planning, and their support of the project should be sought. Users can be included through an advisory committee or through focus groups held early in the planning process. User group composition can include faculty, researchers, professionals, and students. The group may be purely advisory to the library director or project manager; it can also be charged with oversight of the project for the administration of the institution.

2. *Computing/data communications staff:* Even though the library may have its own systems staff, the growing needs of the electronic library should be discussed with the institution's computer and communications staff. Power requirements, access to internal and external communications networks such as the Internet, local area networks, microcomputing needs, and a host of other information technologies must be addressed. These changeable electronic requirements will necessitate the utmost in flexibility to allow the addition of cables or wires to provide convenient locations for future needs. The expertise of this staff in the prediction of future trends is invaluable.

3. *Facilities management staff:* Most large organizations have a facilities planning department which includes architects, engineers, construction managers, electricians, and others. This department may be responsible for carrying out the planning and construction of the new library or for renovations. A project manager from this department may act in a capacity similar to the project manager in the library, in which case the two should work very closely and communicate often. The facilities team will deal with important issues such as fire safety and security that may have an impact on the final design. The engineering staff also will work closely with the architects, construction contractors, and subcontractors. Development of a good rapport with these partners will allow library planners to monitor progress, problems, and/or changes in the building plans during construction.

Selection of Architects

It is vital that a representative of the library be involved in the selection of the architectural firm. In most instances, choosing the firm rests in the hands of some other group in the university or hospital, such as facilities management or procurement; however, the library should take an active role in the selection process. The library's project manager may participate in the early stage of the selection process, the review of responses to a request for proposals from competing firms. The object of the review of these proposals is to develop a short list of architectural firms for further consideration. To make this review process as fair as possible, many institutions construct evaluation grids with points assigned to specific criteria. Some of the evaluation elements include the following elements:

- *Credentials of the architectural firms:* How large is the firm? Is it a nationally recognized firm? Does it have any local expertise? Where did the architects receive their education and training? Have individuals or the firm received awards or recognition for their work? A résumé for each individual proposed for the project should be included.
- *Expertise:* Has the firm been involved in similar projects? Does it have areas of expertise that would be useful to the project?
- *Lead architect:* Who in the firm will be involved? Does the design team that is being proposed include principals of the firm or is much of the work to be done by junior associates?
- *Current workload:* Does the firm have enough time and staff to devote to the project?
- *Team composition:* Who else does the architectural firm propose as part of the team of mechanical and electrical engineers, structural engineers, geotechnical experts, interior designers, lighting and acoustical specialists, and library consultants. What are their credentials and backgrounds? If a library consultant is proposed, the library participant on the selection committee may prove particularly useful because the library community is small and many consultants may be well known based on their publications, professional expertise, and stature in the library community.
- *A sampling and explanation of relevant former projects:* Can the architect demonstrate pertinent experience designing similar facilities?
- *References:* Have prior clients been satisfied with the architect's work and the way in which client needs were addressed?

When the initial review process is complete, references usually are checked, and the list is narrowed to a smaller number of firms that will be invited to prepare a presentation. It is a good idea to involve as many people as can be accommodated for presentations. Top library administration, including the director and project manager, and representation from the institution and constituent groups should be included. This may include representatives from facilities management, key departments or schools, students, and other institutional staff that might have an interest in the building, such as the institutional development or fund-raising organizations.

The session usually consists of a presentation by the architects to describe their expertise, interest in, and ideas for the project. Conceptual models may be included, and there should be plenty of time for questions and answers. Metcalf enumerates fourteen points for consideration in selecting an architect [17]:

1. Professional competence and licensing
2. Ability to interpret and understand the needs of the client
3. Imagination and creative ability to supply a unique and satisfactory design in response to the program
4. Good listening skills and the ability to explain clearly the architect's point of view
5. Understanding of the client institution, its standards, problems, and educational objectives
6. An understanding that the primary task is to address the client's functional and esthetical needs
7. Good taste and ability to harmonize functional requirements with the exterior design
8. Good financial estimator and manager
9. Readily available engineering competence (which is particularly important due to the technological needs of libraries today)
10. Willingness to consult with others to bring in additional expertise when needed; a good problem solver
11. Knows how to staff the project appropriately
12. Infinite patience
13. Willingness to learn; keeps an open mind
14. Personal and professional integrity

Although many of these attributes may seem difficult to determine from a presentation, it is possible to get an impression based on responses to questions and the apparent interest of the architectural team. A vision for the project and a level of excitement should be evident. Useful information can be gained from observing the interactions among the presenters. Is the assembled team comfortable with each other? Have they worked together before? Are there prima donnas in the group? Do they show consideration for each other's opinions and ideas? If they don't, will they show consideration for those of their clients? Any discomfort with or doubt at all about the proposed architectural team should signal the need for rejection. Remember that this is a relationship that will last for many years. In discussions with other members of the selection team, library participants must voice opinions concerning the presentations. The opinion of the library representatives should carry as much weight as those of facilities management or other groups since they represent the owners of the building.

Fee Negotiation

In many institutions, library staff may not be involved in fee negotiation as this falls within the purview of a procurement department based on strict guidelines established by the institution or funding agency. However, this is a very important phase and a very interesting process to observe. Architects' fees vary from project to project, from firm to firm, and from institution to institution. These fees are often a percentage of the construction costs. The usual services performed by the architect include the architectural concept and planning of the building, engineering services for structural, plumbing, heating, ventilation, and air-conditioning, and the electrical work [18]. Additional fees may be included to cover the cost of special consultants that need to be involved, including computer professionals, acoustical engineers, or lighting experts. Architectural services are divided into three groups [19]:

1. Preliminary services, which include planning conferences to determine scope of work, schematic design, sketches of proposed design and engineering alternatives, and preliminary cost estimates
2. Construction documents and specifications the contractors will use to construct the building
3. Execution of work, or oversight of the execution of the project

During the fee negotiation process, the architect and a negotiation team go through several rounds of give and take to arrive at a satisfactory cost. To achieve a lower fee, the scope of the project may need to be reduced, which would cause the negotiation team to come back to the library administration to ask whether there are programmatic areas that can be reduced or eliminated. The architects also study their costs and cut and realign where necessary. For example, in the original fee submittal, the architect may have proposed an interior design firm. Upon closer examination, to cut costs, they may decide that their own firm has enough expertise to handle interior design issues, and the interior design firm may be dropped. However, it is very important for the library director or project manager to be consulted if any programmatic changes are proposed. In the worst-case scenario, if a fee cannot be negotiated with the architectural firm, negotiations may be broken off and then begun with the second-choice firm.

Program Verification

After the fees have been negotiated, it is the architect's responsibility to get to know the client and to understand the needs of the program to begin suggesting architectural solutions. In many cases, as discussed earlier, an extensive building program will have been written by the institution. However, if this step has not occurred, the architect may now need to write that program. Through meetings with the client, the architect gains the following information [20]:

- *Objectives and priorities:* What are the expectations of the library administration and of the institution for this building?
- *Personnel forecasts:* How many people will this building house the day it opens? In five years? In ten years?
- *Functional requirements:* What does this building need to do to be successful and meet the expectations of staff, administration, and the institution? What functions will be housed in this building?
- *Space standards:* Does the institution have space requirements, allocations based on functions, or restrictions concerning the amount of space for different services or people?
- *Adjacencies:* What needs to be located where for the building to serve its users and to provide staff with efficient working conditions?

Because both the client and the architect want the project to be a success, much can be gained by successful dialogue and collaboration during these information-gathering sessions. However, as with any new relationship, communication is not always open and forthcoming. Clients may be

reluctant to be decisive, judgmental, and vocal for fear of appearing naive, ignorant, or intrusive. Sometimes architects seem to be equally reluctant to draw out a client and delve into the nitty-gritty of the library's pragmatic needs for fear of appearing less than all-knowing [21].

This type of thinking must be eradicated.

One method for collaborative planning that works very successfully is known as *wallboarding*. In a wallboarding session, all input is captured on large pieces of newsprint and hung around the planning room. As discussions evolve, information is recorded and reworked, but the history of the ideas and interactions remains on the wall. A similar planning technique is called *charette* [22]. Both share ground rules and outcomes. The object is to break down communications barriers and explore ideas, feelings, and goals. These meetings are informal and set for a focused period of time, and all parties work toward agreed-on goals in a mutually respectful climate. During some wallboarding sessions, the staff is invited to review the work in progress and record their questions or comments directly on the wallboards. By the end of these sessions, the architects and the clients reach agreement on the basic elements for schematic design. According to Michael [23], wall-boarding or charette sessions offer the following advantages:

- An opportunity to discuss elements of and issues in library architecture, which can be very educational for the library client
- Development of enthusiasm and commitment when the creative ideas begin to flow freely and people dream of what might be
- Opportunities for many to explain their goals, dreams, needs, and concerns, which enhances a sense of empowerment and inclusion
- Unforeseen design opportunities that begin to come to light along with options that may not have been included within the program plan
- Bonding among the members of the team—architects, clients, engineers, and consultants
- An appreciation for the skills of the architects and designers, and the thrill of seeing designs and graphic representations of ideas

Whatever the methodology, after gathering this information, the architect begins to piece together the library puzzle. With this knowledge and with information regarding the site and its constraints, the architect makes some preliminary suggestions concerning the way the building should be placed on the site and the way interior elements should be placed to accomplish desired adjacencies and functions. A number of different scenarios may be suggested to test certain solutions and to clarify and verify the client's preferences. This whole process requires open dialogue, suggestions, and give and take between the architect and client.

Schematic Design

The schematic design phase further refines the program. After gathering data and verifying programmatic needs, the architect begins to design a building that meets institutional needs within the square footage and the site constraints. Structural, mechanical, and electrical engineers are brought in to aid in the process by studying the feasibility of the proposed configurations. The architect looks at the practical and aesthetic possibilities for the exterior of the building, and the design begins to evolve. The interior spaces emerge based on square footage allocations and function. Major public elements such as entrances, elevators, stairs, and service desks are placed. Many library staff should review the progress near the end of the schematic design phase. A number of different designs may be presented, and by the end of this phase, the architect and the librarians should be in agreement concerning general concepts for the building and its layout. When all concerns have been answered satisfactorily, the next phase commences.

Design Development

The design development phase focuses on the details of the building design. The exterior elevations will be finalized, but the detail work concentrates on the interior. Final wall placements occur, and an interior designer interviews staff and designs the collection, staff, and user spaces. This may involve drawing office layouts and selecting a conceptual model for the furnishings. Individual departments may be asked to meet with the architectural team to discuss workflow within their units and to identify optimal layouts. An active exchange of information satisfies the needs of both groups. The burden falls to the client to communicate all requirements and to make it known whether a proposal is unsatisfactory. Once construction has started, it is much harder and more costly to change things.

During design development, the architectural team will also work on the final layouts for shelving, lounge seating, service areas, study rooms, classrooms, and computer rooms. Many detailed questions need to be asked and answered. In addition to layouts, the architectural team will work on the interior finishes, such as selecting colors and wall finishes, grades of carpeting, trim work, windows, and window coverings. As the design becomes more detailed, so do the drawings. A good working knowledge of reading blueprints is necessary. At the end of design development, a much larger set of blueprints will be submitted, and, as at the end of schematic design, there will be a review period for client approval. These very thorough documents must be reviewed closely, although major issues should have been resolved earlier in the process. Review in design development focuses on double-checking that earlier suggestions have been incorporated and on adding final detailed design elements. This is another good time to involve staff in the review process, especially where it involves their functional areas. With acceptance of the design development documents, the preparation of construction documents begins.

Construction Documents

Construction documents delineate in great detail how the building will be built. They may include, but are not limited to, landscape design, the exterior elevations, interior plans, furniture layouts, interior finishes such as door hardware and floor coverings, electrical plans, computing and communications details such as wiring, mechanical systems including heating and air-conditioning, plumbing, details of built-ins such as service desks, lighting, and security systems. An intense review of these documents may involve a large team with members responsible for particular sections of the documents based on expertise. Drawings may be submitted at a 50%, or halfway, phase and a 90% or 95% phase to make sure that the documents proceed without significant misconceptions or errors.

Upon completion of the review of the construction documents, they form the base from which to bid out the project for construction. The institutional procurement office sends out an invitation to bid, and construction companies respond. Frequently, the project is awarded to the lowest bidder who meets the technical terms of the construction requirements. Although there may be little that the library project manager can contribute to the technical evaluation, it is important to participate in the interview of the construction firm for many of the same reasons given previously for assessing the architects.

With the construction firm selected, responsibility for overseeing the project will probably fall to an institution's facilities or architecture and engineering groups who will usually assign their own project manager. It is important to establish a relationship with this project manager and have good and open lines of communication so that the library's influence continues during the crucial construction phase. At this time it may be a good idea to acquire a hard hat and heavy work boots!

The construction project manager and the construction superintendent constitute the two main contacts from the construction firm. The construction project manager oversees the progress of the project and manages much of the paperwork. The construction superintendent oversees the subcontractors and the actual fieldwork of constructing the building. On smaller projects this one person may fulfill both roles. Regular construction progress meetings and site walks should occur in which the library project manager demonstrates interest in the project, raises questions or asks for clarification, and demonstrates accessibility. It is important to note that just as the library project manager is the single route of communication for gathering and disseminating information from the library planning groups, the institutional project manager fills the same function for the construction phase. All major communications regarding any changes, modifications, or opinions should be conveyed through that person.

SPACE PLANNING

Planning a library for the twenty-first century is a daunting task with many uncertainties and pitfalls. At the same time, it poses an exciting challenge. Can the librarian envision how information will be stored and retrieved in twenty years or how users will access that information? Such planning requires that technology be integrated into the full range of work and services found in a library. The success of a library building is measured by how well it serves both the users and the staff, by how effective and efficient it is. To this end it must facilitate users' access to information through the library's services and both print and electronic collections, and it must allow efficient use of staff resources.

What constitutes an effective and efficient library building? Habich states that "effective and efficient library buildings result from synergistic meshing of form and function" [24]. An effective library building anticipates user needs and expectations. Its configuration creates patterns logical to the user and should be self-explanatory. A user should not have to search for assistance but readily see where service points exist. Cues to a building's effective use include (1) an easily accessible entrance from the main traffic paths; (2) readily accessible high-use areas, such as those for the online catalog and other electronic resources; (3) highly visible service and staff points; and (4) logical arrangement of the collection [25].

A well-designed library embodies both architectural and operational efficiency. Specific elements include

- a high ratio of net (usable) to gross square footage,
- low operating costs,
- modular design,
- functional area locations that minimize steps for staff and users,
- high-use areas near the entrance,
- fixed building elements that do not intrude,
- related service points that are physically close to each other, and
- service point locations that allow flexible staffing for peak and off-peak hours [26].

Overall the building should be flexible enough to accommodate changes in technology.

Planning for Technology

It is appropriate at this point to highlight the impact of technology on library design and space planning. Older formulas for collection growth and space requirements for users and staff no longer apply. Although it may seem impossible to plan for evolving technology, the infrastructure of the building and the overall space must be flexible over time.

Collaboration between the institutional telecommunications staff and library systems staff is crucial. Together they will meet with electrical engineers to design an infrastructure that supports current and future services. The planning and infrastructure design occurs on two levels, one very pragmatic and one more visionary. On a pragmatic level, it is important to determine where conduit will run. Should it go only to specific areas, or should it undergird the entire structure? The visionary planning concerns what wiring will run in the conduit. What are the current institutional standards? Are these standards adequate for a library with its increasing support of full-text graphics, video, and audio? Will the infrastructure include hubs and routers, or will it be a switched network with direct connections to networks? Must the electrical grid in the building support wireless communication?

Space Configuration

The site will determine the shape of a library unless there happens to be a large open space. The site can be long and narrow, on a hillside, in a cramped area, or in part of another building. Architects recommend either a square or a rectangle not more than twice as long as it is wide as the ideal. Hitt points out features to be avoided, such as a long narrow floor, several small floors, interior walls, mezzanines, and curved or angled walls [27].

Size

How many square feet should be allocated for various functions? As mentioned earlier, the impact of technology lessened the usefulness of formulas traditionally employed in space planning. Space planning in the past generally addressed only user seats, collections, and staff. Space planning has become more complicated and must consider service areas that include the reference and circulation desks, computer workstations for users, wired carrels, classrooms to teach computer use and information management, wired group study rooms, and possibly distance learning facilities. The library of the future needs to accommodate these and other new resources and services. Additionally, print books and electronic media will to some extent replace journals. To make matters worse, staff workspace needs change as technologies evolve.

Collection Space Needs

Estimating the square footage that will be required to house a collection for the next twenty to thirty years is indeed difficult. Metcalf provides a thorough discussion of stacks and shelving [28]; however, he warns that, "[i]f a completely satisfactory formula could be provided for such estimates, the task would be greatly simplified, but experience suggests rather that the first rule should be Beware of Formulas" [29].

Collection growth can be projected in several ways: (1) use a standard 4% per year compounded approach, (2) aim at a specific collection size, and (3) assume that local average growth over the past few years will continue into the future [30]. The first approach assumes a predictable budget, which in these days of shrinking library resources is probably best avoided. The second could work in a collection such as a hospital library, where generally only current materials will be required and regular weeding is done. In the third approach, the average growth of each format for the last five years is calculated and that figure is multiplied by the number of years in the planning period.

Two notes of caution: First, conservatism suggests adding about five years to the normal twenty-year planning cycle used for libraries, especially in publicly funded institutions. The time between writing the program and actually occupying the building could be five to ten years since the request and funding process can be lengthy. Second, look at the goals of your particular library in terms of electronic resources. Anticipate a slower rate of print growth as more journals are published electronically. One way to deal with this uncertainty is to build flexibility into stack areas, allowing future conversion to user workspace for accessing electronic media. Unfortunately, no formula has been developed to make realistic projections regarding the ratio of print to electronic collection growth.

Once the collection size for which space will be required has been established, a number of important questions remain. For example, to how many bound volume equivalents (BVEs) does this convert? How many BVEs are in a linear foot of shelving (books and journals), and, based on this figure, how many ranges of what size are needed? How much square footage is required for stacks that shelve the collections? To what working capacity should shelves be filled? There are a number of approaches to answering these questions; Metcalf [31], Fraley and Anderson [32], and Hitt [33] provide thorough discussions.

The following example illustrates how inexact space projections can be. In Maryland the state's four-year public college and university space-planning guidelines and the Association of College and Research Libraries (ACRL) standard were compared and then modified to project the growth of electronic versus print collections. The 1995 ACRL standards recommend the following area for stack space:

For the first 150,000 volumes:	0.10 square feet/volume
For the next 150,000 volumes:	0.09 square feet/volume
For the next 300,000 volumes:	0.08 square feet/volume
Over 600,000 volumes:	0.07 square feet/volume

Applying this formula to a library holding 400,000 volumes results in a stack space requirement of 36,500 square feet. By comparison, the Maryland state guidelines call for the following areas:

1 to 150,000 medical volumes:	0.15 square feet/volume
Over 150,000 medical volumes:	0.12 square feet/volume
All volumes in general collections:	0.08 square feet/volume

The UMBC health sciences library collection can be divided into medical science materials, which account for approximately 60%, and social science materials, which account for 40% of the volumes. Applying the state formula to a library containing 400,000 volumes with a 60/40 split results in a stack space requirement of 44,600 square feet. This is 22% more space than the ACRL formula provides.

Table 6-1 projects the future space requirements for stack space as the UMBC collection size increases as calculated from the Maryland guidelines. Based on these considerations and the continued use of compact shelving for older materials, it was proposed that 45,970 square feet be made available for UMBC library stacks and storage of other information media [34].

One alternative for calculating the square footage needed to house the collection is to apply the *cubook formula*, which specifies that a square foot of floor space will house ten volumes at working capacity [35]. In short, this would mean that a collection of 400,000 volumes requires 40,000 square feet for stack space. One must also define when the stack is considered at full working capacity, with advice ranging from 66% [36] to 86% full [37]. Whatever percentage is chosen, enough space must be left to shift collections and reshelve comfortably. Several other elements affect the allocation of space as well: (1) range spacing and lengths, (2) aisle widths as mandated by the Americans with Disabilities Act (ADA), (3) the number of cross aisles and their widths, (4) the number of structural columns and their placement, and (5) the number of shelves per section [38]. Other areas of stacks and shelving that require special consideration are described next.

Reference Stacks

Both staff and users make heavy use of reference stacks. Hitt states that a large academic health sciences library should accommodate 8,000 to 10,000 reference volumes and have wider than normal aisles [39]. Moreover, shelves should not obstruct the view of the room from the reference desk. Thought should be given to how these volumes are best used, either in consulting areas interspersed throughout the stacks or on the periphery of the area. If the shelves are low enough for books to be placed on them, the tops should be a durable material. Traditionally, tables for the most heavily used indexes

Table 6-1: Projected Stack Space Requirements by Maryland State Guidelines

Year	Total Collection Size (Volumes)	BVE	Square Feet Required
2000	409,100	531,830	45,546
2005	459,100	596,830	50,746
2010	509,100	661,830	55,946

and abstracts are included in the reference area. In planning for the future, however, it is important to consider that many of these tools are now searched electronically and fewer tables may be needed.

Current Journal Stacks

A variety of shelving systems are available for current journals. Some libraries choose to have all current journals in one area and in alphabetical order. This simplifies access for the user. Other schemes have only a specific subset of journals in this area. Many titles that are considered serials, such as reference titles and monographic series, generally are not placed in current journal stacks in a health sciences library. Some libraries may also wish to have a special display of current titles, such as those received each day or week. This requires more sophisticated monitoring by staff and requires additional space, possibly in a reference or lounge area.

Rare Book Stacks

Depending on the size of the collection, two types of rare book stacks may be planned—one for display purposes and another for preservation. Since the rare book room often serves as a showplace for the library, some stacks may be built-in, wooden cases with glass or mesh locked doors. These can be in a comfortable rare book reading room that exhibits nonfragile works. If the collection is large enough, a climate-controlled, windowless stack area should be built to house various types of materials including books, manuscripts, or photographs needing long-term preservation. Usually, the public will not be admitted to this area, but materials to be consulted would be brought to them in the rare book reading room.

Compact Shelving

Compact shelving maximizes collection storage space, usually doubling storage capacity. Most often it is used to forestall additions to library buildings or new buildings, but it can also be part of the collection space planning in a new facility. Structural considerations should not be overlooked because the floor must be able to handle 300 pounds per square foot, as opposed to the normal 150 pounds per square foot for regular shelving [40]. Compact shelving choices include manually or electronically operated systems. Electrical compact shelving has special installation requirements for wiring and power sources. Whichever type is selected, lighting and traffic patterns must also be considered. Careful thought should be given to whether the material shelved there will be high or low use and whether access will be open to the public or staff only. Both Metcalf [41] and Fraley and Anderson [42] detail the advantages and disadvantages of compact shelving.

Public Space Needs

Peters discusses seating space for library users in a digital era [43]. Various formulas exist to project the number of seats based on the number of faculty, staff, and student full-time equivalents (FTEs) at the institution, but these must be questioned because of the electronic revolution. If information is readily accessible on the World Wide Web at one's own desk, many administrators ask how much the institution should invest in reader space. Providing support to networked information resources is a primary function of the library and should be a major consideration in designing library facilities. It requires a fresh look at service points, instructional facilities, individual and group study areas, and "docking stations" where users can plug in their own laptops to access and/or manipulate information.

Seating Space Requirements

Current space requirements for seating generally are based on the total number of clients served. States and institutions may have their own formulas that they prefer to use, but ACRL guidelines recommend one reading seat for every five primary users and twenty-five to thirty-five square feet for each, depending on use [44]. Based on a user population of 8,100, for example, with thirty square feet per user station, ACRL calls for 48,600 net square feet. The state or university guideline may be more complex. For example, the state of Maryland uses a formula that allocates seating for proportions of the population of each user category: undergraduate FTEs are assigned thirty square feet, while graduate students and faculty are assigned forty square feet. Square footage may need to be adjusted to reflect other factors, such as the commuting nature of a campus.
In 1994 Henshaw pointed out:

> There does not exist a documented body of knowledge relative to the design of the library of the future. Much of the knowledge accumulated over the past one hundred years regarding successful library design isn't applicable to the current situation [45].

Contrary to modern myths about the declining popularity of the library as a facility, use has actually increased during the last decade. Electronic access allows users to identify more materials more easily, which in turn increases the demand for print documents. Moreover, the demand for instructional services in the use of the Internet and electronic resources has grown dramatically over the last several years. The shift to problem-based learning curricula places even more importance on library print, electronic, and instructional resources.

Types of Seating

Different user purposes will require a mix of carrels, group study rooms, tables, public access workstations, classrooms (including distance education and microcomputer), and lounge areas. Users continue to enjoy sunlit reader spaces around the perimeter of the floor with books protected in stacks placed away from damaging ultraviolet rays.

Carrels

Study carrels can be purchased from a library furniture vendor or can be custom built. Carrels should have enough space to house a computer or other electronic equipment as well as print materials the reader may be using at the same time. Effective lighting is important to be able to support reading both print and electronic media. In some carrels wiring should be present for required electricity and data communication connections. The inclusion of a depressed space or pull-out tray for computer keyboards may be desired in some settings.

Group Study Rooms

As alluded to earlier, the need for group study and collaboration has become quite important for problem-based curricula. Rooms should be able to accommodate between six and eight persons as well as table, chairs, and possibly a shelf for electronic equipment. Each room should have a whiteboard, be soundproof, provide glare protection from windows, and have a partial glass door or wall for security purposes. In planning for the future, it also is essential to provide the wiring and conduit for access to electronic resources.

Tables

Except in conference rooms, tables that seat more than four people are to be avoided. Usually only one or two people will sit at a table even if it can seat more. Tables are appropriate for readers who have materials to spread out and for areas where carrels are too obstructive. Tables can now be obtained that have openings or conduit to house wiring for persons bringing their own computer, which necessitates planning for the location and availability of wiring. Privacy and noise control are additional challenges.

Public Access Workstations

Most libraries now provide public workstations to access electronic resources such as the online catalog, databases, or word-processing software. Many libraries have "shoe-horned" these stations into existing facilities near the reference service area where assistance is available. In planning a new facility, it remains important to locate these tools near a service point. Additional stations may be on other floors where materials are located. The station should comfortably accommodate the computer, printer, books, a work surface to write on, and a chair, often thirty-five to forty square feet per station. It may be a good idea to cluster them in groups of four to give a more practical arrangement and more pleasing visual impression.

Classroom

In referring to microcomputing classrooms in 1988, Hitt stated that "[t]he planning team should give serious thought to the space and the security required for this new library service" [46]. Twelve years later, the teaching role of the librarian has become well established. Facilities for instruction, which were almost an afterthought in earlier library design, are now central to the library's mission. Instructional facilities support access to the full range of electronic media and instructional methodologies. Looming large on the horizon is the need to support distance learning, with the library a likely location for such a facility. Ideally, classrooms should accommodate between twelve and twenty-four workstations with thirty to thirty-five square feet for each. Each station should be similar to the public access workstation described above. However, for some types of instruction, whiteboards, screens, and projectors should also be available in the room.

Staff and Service Space Needs

Planning space for staff and service areas requires a good grasp of functional relationships—in other words, how the library works. Normally, functional relationships are examined carefully during the schematic design phase. In doing so, one not only looks at existing relationships, functions, and the organizational structure but also anticipates how these might change in the future. Bubble diagrams and flowcharting may be useful in analyzing proximity of staff to each other and of staff to service areas.

Planning typically reviews the following types of questions:

1 What functions should be close to the entrance?
2. Where should staff offices and work areas be in relation to service points?
3. Should staff work areas be near the reference and electronic access areas?
4. Where should interlibrary loan and document delivery be in relation to stacks? To circulation?
5. Should the systems staff be near microcomputer classrooms?
6. Does the library director wish to be near the entrance or farther from the public eye?
7. Should staff areas be grouped around an elevator?
8. What departments need to be near each other? Do they require horizontal or vertical adjacencies?

Staff Space Requirements

Most guides to library planning suggest that between 20% and 25% of the total reader and collection space is needed for staff [47-48], yet it is difficult to anticipate the size of the staff twenty years hence. Although some past authors argued that automation would reduce staff size, this has not been the reality. Staff has simply been shifted from technical processing to systems or public services. Likewise, the advent of end user searching has not reduced staff but has shifted staff from searching to training functions. Although it may be difficult to justify, more space should be requested for staff than in the current facility. If it is a larger facility, more staff will be needed to provide services. Experience also bears out that staff space usually suffers first as space begins to run out. Staff should be provided with a pleasant work environment because they spend more time in the library than anyone else. Resist the architect who wants to relegate staff to basement, windowless spaces!

Some planning techniques call for estimates of future staffing levels for each department and by type of position. The space allocated to each individual must include all requirements, such as desks, files, computer workstations, book trucks, consultation or conference tables, copiers, or fax machines. Most likely there are state guidelines for allocating staff space. For example, the Maryland and other state space planning guidelines provide 150 square feet for individual private offices. Private offices should be insisted on for directors, division heads, department heads, and others such as personnel officers or budget administrators who deal with sensitive personnel or financial data.

Planning for Technology in Libraries

Marks states that users of high-technology equipment, both staff and patrons, too often receive "short shrift" in the planning process.

Confining a library staff member to 50, 75, or even 125 square feet may create an intolerable work environment. . . . Influencing the square footage needed for an adequate work space will be the set of factors that are encompassed by the term ergonomic. . . . A work space should be large enough to accommodate a workstation that has the computer screen positioned so that the user looks down at an angle of fifteen to twenty degrees. The eye-to-screen distance for the user should be twenty to thirty-five inches. If the individual is working with copy, it should be held at the same height as the screen. The work surface on which the workstation is located should be adjustable so that the keyboard is about thirty inches from the floor. This will allow the person's upper arms to hang vertically and the forearms to angle downward slightly. This presumes there is a chair with five casters and an adjustable seat height of fifteen to twenty-one inches above the floor, with an adjustable backrest to support the small of the back. All furniture should be certified as nonstatic and chairs or tables with casters should be lubricated with graphite. A cramped work space will not allow an ergonomically effective arrangement of the equipment to be achieved [49].

Office landscaping or modular furniture offers an effective way to manage staff space. This allows flexibility in arrangement and design of the space and the furniture. Staff should be afforded privacy with enough space to house required equipment or materials. For efficient work flow, enough space should be allowed to move among personal workspaces. Office landscape design should incorporate shared equipment and space for fax machines, copiers, or files and a meeting area. On the negative side, modular panels can block access to electrical or network jacks and can impede air flow.

Nonpublic Staff Spaces

Behind-the-scenes library functions form the foundation for all the public services, and as such, the space for this staff is critical.

Access Services

The circulation desk often presents the busiest, noisiest, and most congested area in the library. The staff area, however, is also a beehive of behind-the-scenes activity. Space allocation depends on the size of the library and the services offered by circulation staff. In many cases, students or part-time staff are hired who do not require the same level of space or shift workers may share space. The types of activities that may be considered for staff space allocation include reserve materials preparation including scanning for electronic reserve systems; sorting books for reshelving; checking in books; collection of fine money; sale of products such as copy cards or diskettes; photocopying services; fax receiving and transmitting. In addition to terminals at the desk, equipment needs may include microcomputers for staff, fax machines, scanners, photocopiers, book trucks, a safe for money, a cash register, and lockers for part-time staff.

An important staff function is monitoring security for the collection. Circulation staff normally respond to the alarm at the entry or possibly at fire exit doors or stairs. Some libraries choose to have a security system panel installed behind the desk that can be monitored by staff. Placement of this setup should be convenient so that it can be observed during times of low staffing. Circulation staff normally open and close the library, and they need access to lighting controls.

Administration

While the administration offices need not be on the main floor, they should be easily accessible by the public and staff. The director should certainly have a private office in any size library. Additional office space for a receptionist, secretary, administrative aide, or personnel officer may also be required. Space for office equipment and files seems always to be in short supply. If the administrative staff is large, office landscaping is preferred for support staff.

Information and Instructional Services

As a key service area in the library, this space must be planned with great care. Important questions include the following:

- Should the information/reference staff area be open to the public?
- Should the staff have private offices, or will office landscaping do?
- What type of instructional materials preparation area is needed?
- What type of equipment will each individual need? The group?
- How close to the reference desk or computer searching area should they be?
- Is a separate room needed for consultation services?

Computer and other electronic equipment will become ever more important, especially as the educational and instructional role of the library increases. Space and power needs for specialized equipment such as scanners should be allocated as well.

Public services staff should be heavily involved in making decisions about their workspace. Many believe they should be in close proximity to user areas because it is easier for clients to find help. Other staff believe the constant interruptions do not allow them the appropriate time to work on projects, solve information problems, or develop the quality instructional materials they require. Staff should have input on this because it will affect their ability to function well.

Interlibrary Loan/Document Delivery

At the present time, these functions remain paper-intensive, although requests for the material may be sent and received electronically. The volume of these services themselves grows, partly because users have access to more bibliographic information but also because libraries are buying less and depending on others to provide more material. However, direct user access to full-text information may change this in the future. This said, for now the space must house the staff as well as quite a variety of equipment. The planner must also understand whether the unit is part of reference, technical services, or circulation and whether borrowing and lending operations are split. Does the staff deal directly with the public? Ideally, how close to the stacks should the staff be?

Resources Management

Many libraries call this area "Technical Services," and it includes cataloging, acquisitions, serials control, and binding. Some libraries include collection development, interlibrary loan, and stack maintenance as well. The functions of this group can be accommodated well by office landscaping that reflects the flow to materials being processed. Proximity to the shipping and receiving area is vital for this staff, through either horizontal or vertical adjacency. The workstation for each staff member must accommodate computer equipment as well as a work surface for the materials being processed. Additionally, book trucks, shelving, storage space, and any other equipment needed by all staff should be in a conveniently located spot. For libraries using online catalogs, little or no space is now needed for card files! Binding personnel may require large tables and other specialized equipment as well as a fully functional sink.

Systems

A large library may have from one to five or more systems staff, and may add more over time. Generally speaking, it does not matter where systems staff is located although, if they support a computing assistance desk, it is desirable to have offices located close by. Noise and temperature may make it impractical to put staff in the same room with the computers, but it is efficient to have them nearby. Staff need sufficient workspace for daily operations, and to test new products, store equipment and documentation, and do in-house repair work. We strongly recommend that systems staff be given a maximum of space. Experience shows that obsolete and broken equipment, documentation, and new equipment quickly usurp large amounts of storage space.

Other Nonpublic Spaces

Conference Rooms

The need for conference rooms is based on the size of the library staff and the availability of the room to others. In a small library, the library director's office may serve as a conference room or have one directly connected to it. At least one room should be large enough for the senior administrative team to meet. If the library is large, more than one room may be needed so that departments, task forces, or committees have a space to meet. Because there never seems to be enough meeting space, it is wise to plan for conference rooms that can be used for other purposes, such as small classrooms. If the library plans to make its conference room available to others, it should be visible and accessible from a public area. Some libraries use conference rooms for special occasions such as receptions, which then requires adjacent space for food preparation, storage of extra furniture, and coats.

In general, a conference room should seat between ten and thirty people comfortably. One or more tables or a table that can be taken apart should be provided along with appropriate chairs. Power and wiring, as well as space for a projection screen, computer equipment, whiteboards, and storage will be needed. If the room has windows, appropriate window coverings should be installed to be able to darken the room.

Staff Lounge

The staff lounge serves as an extremely important a place for informal meetings, staff celebrations, or just eating lunch. Metcalf suggests ten to fifteen square feet for each FTE staff member [50]. In a large library, a basic kitchen and lounge and eating area should be included. Essentials include a sink with garbage disposal, refrigerator(s), microwave, and coffee makers. A mix of tables and chairs as well as some sofas and stuffed chairs should be provided. The staff lounge should either be away from public areas or entered only by key or access panel to ensure privacy.

Mail Room/Loading Dock

This receiving area must accommodate deliveries coming into the library, deliveries from the mailroom to other library areas, and all outgoing mail. Hitt advises that a receiving room's delivery entrance must be easily accessible and totally secure from unauthorized entrance or exit, allow for truck access, and protect materials and personnel from inclement weather. An external bell, buzzer, or telephone is required to announce delivery. Double doors to the loading dock and into the building interior are needed for furniture and large equipment. Wide items also mandate spacious corridors. The receiving function may take place via a workroom or technical services space, but every effort should be made to avoid deliveries coming through the main entrance because users may be inconvenienced and public areas could become damaged. Hitt further advises:

> As in planning for all spaces in the library, make sure all receiving-room functions are allowed for. Incoming and outgoing mail, including bindery shipments, will be processed here. A sink, work tables, postage machines, wrapping materials and considerable floor space to house large shipments temporarily are all implied. The receiving room is also the ideal place for the storage of library supplies; a wall of single-faced shelving with 12" shelves is a good solution. The author has yet to see a new health science library with enough storage space. Do all you can to make the receiving room as large as possible, for inevitably it will need to be used partly for storage purposes [51].

Storage Space

Plan as much storage space as possible for each department in the library. No one has ever complained of too much storage! Not only are there general supplies, paper for photocopiers, printers, forms, pamphlets, and materials produced by the library but also old or extra furniture, spare or broken computer equipment, boxes of gift books, and display material. If you have difficulty getting storage space into your plans, call it something else that is acceptable, but be sure you have it!

Conservation and Exhibit Preparation Space

These two areas may have a low priority. Space can be included in Resources Management or the historical collections area in larger libraries. Staff will need a large table, some storage cabinets for materials, and, if possible, a sink with running water.

Public Service Spaces

The foregoing section discussed questions and considerations in planning nonpublic staff spaces. This section will address the issues to consider in planning the public services spaces not covered earlier.

Lobby/Entry

An impressive lobby or entry to the library can set the tone for the building. It should invite, illuminate, and be as spacious as possible. Clutter and dimness are to be avoided along with the impulse to put every bit of information right by the door. Try to draw users from the door to the information inside the building. Many libraries will have a security system to control entry and exit and, in some cases, a guard who sits at a desk to check identification. The circulation desk must allow quick access to the entry if a problem occurs there. It is a good idea to have automatic doors so users can enter and exit easily. Such doors also meet requirements for access by clients with disabilities.

Circulation Service Desk

The circulation desk often appears to be the center of activity in the library. The overall size of the library, the services offered, and the number of users will determine the size and shape of the desk. There are six essentials to remember when designing this important desk [52]:

1. The desk should be of a size that can accommodate several staff conducting business at the same time, but not so large that one person alone cannot manage at low-use times.
2. There should be space for users to put down the books they want to charge out; there should be a book drop or slot for books being returned.
3. Terminals should be placed below the top level to avoid wire clutter and provide more space for the user. Two-tier desks can be designed to accommodate terminals, barcode readers, and other essentials.
4. Space should be designed for a cash register. In addition to collecting overdue fines, circulation may be the spot to pick up and pay for other services, such as interlibrary loan, photocopy, or search results.

5. The desk top should be as durable as possible because it probably will get more wear than any other surface in the library. The length, shape, width, and height should be considered carefully as the desk should not only be efficient and functional, but having a pleasing appearance as well. One section should be low enough to meet ADA requirements.
6. The desk should have space for distributing brochures and forms as well as a place to leave service requests for interlibrary loans and the like.

The circulation staff space should be adjacent and convenient to the desk but generally not immediately behind it. Staff who are working on other tasks will find it difficult to concentrate with the noise of activity, users, equipment, and general traffic.

Information Service Desk

Another major hub of activity in the library is the information/reference service desk. The optimum location for the information service desk is near circulation and the lobby where the user can see it upon entering. In addition to the desk itself, adjacent areas must be planned carefully to house resources or to offer the assistance of an information professional. Areas that should be considered for close proximity to the desk include the ready-reference collection, print indexes and abstracts, workstations to access electronic databases and services and online catalogs, and microform readers. The reference desk should appear welcoming. Avoid the fortress look! Many users are reluctant to seek assistance, and an accessible reference desk may encourage them to ask for help.

Like the circulation desk, this desk should also be uncluttered so that users have space to put their books or papers while talking to staff. Prefer a two-tier type of desk so that workstations and telephones can be placed below the counter. Some libraries may prefer to have a lower section where a client may sit and speak with staff; this also can serve as access for persons with disabilities. Another important aspect of the desk is an opening that allows staff to easily step through to assist people; staff should face both users and resources so that they will be able to oversee the entire area.

Conveniences and Amenities

Numerous conveniences and amenities must be remembered. Their importance will depend on the size and location of the library, whether it is freestanding or within another building.

Photocopiers

No library can exist without these. If the library has more than one floor, it is helpful to locate them in the same area on each floor. A separate room eliminates noise but requires attention to airflow and good ventilation.

Book Drops

Users appreciate book drops outside the library. Consider locations carefully to avoid damage to materials, and consider staff time needed to collect the books.

Vending Areas

Although most libraries try to prohibit food and drink, users will be pleased if a space can be provided for some snacks or drinks. Some libraries promote spillproof containers for beverages that are brought into the library.

Public Telephones

Some public telephones are essential, especially in-house telephones for use by hospital or medical center staff.

Card Vending Machines and Change Machines

Vending machines for copicards or other services may be needed along with a change machine if the library has coin-operated services.

Rest Rooms and Water Fountains

The architect will certainly include these necessities. Be sure that locations are convenient, visible, and predictable for users. Separate facilities for staff should be considered if the library is a large one.

Elevators

A public elevator and a freight elevator will be necessary if the library has more than one floor. The freight elevator should be adjacent to the loading dock or mailroom with the public elevator(s) in or adjacent to the lobby.

Other

The library may want to consider public bulletin boards or information kiosks in a location that minimizes visual clutter. Coat racks, umbrella stands, and lockers are other amenities users appreciate.

CORE ELEMENTS

At this time any discussion of core elements must begin with the technological infrastructure. Those advising a simplistic approach might suggest "wiring the heck out of the building," but much more thought is needed. Although it is important to plan purposefully where all the wiring will go, it may be more important to design a flexible building that can be modified easily in response to rapid changes in information technology [53]. One can maximize flexibility without knowing the exact nature of future functions.

Planning for flexibility can benefit from consideration of thoughtful questions. Are services driving the technology or is technology driving services? What types of services will be provided by this facility? Will there be a central computer facility? What about multipurpose, multimedia workstations that will access databases, the Internet, or graphic images? Will there be training, distance education, or telemedicine facilities in the building? Should the wiring accommodate voice, data, and full-motion video? Do users carry laptops that need docking stations for network connections in carrels or study room? Will staff require high-capacity wiring to the desktop? Do the stack areas need wiring? Will everything be linked via local area networks or use cellular or wireless communications? Are there strict wiring standards within the institution? How will the library be connected to the outside electronic world?

Although these questions seem endless, they are all vital. Many may have been addressed in the building program for the facility. Technology support is expensive but "it will never be any less expensive to install the infrastructure than it is while construction and renovation are occurring" [54]. A major part of the technological infrastructure is electricity. Marks advises that current electrical needs be calculated and then increased by 50% to 100% [55]. Quad outlets as opposed to duplex outlets should be considered for each office wall. All major computing equipment will benefit from uninterrupted power system sources [56].

The conduit size for electrical and cabling needs is critical. Spending a small amount now for larger conduit will avoid the greater cost of installing a second conduit later. Fiber optic cabling does not need to run through conduit. A series of hooks or cable trays can be used to suspend and support cables within the ceilings. Many libraries being planned today employ a three-duct system with one portion of the conduit reserved for telephone cabling, one the electrical wires, and one the data cabling.

Technology also affects environmental conditions such as temperature, humidity, noise, and lighting. A mainframe computer room within the building will require its own air-conditioning and environmental controls. Smaller computers need only room air-conditioning. A humidity level of about 50% controls static [57]. Concentrations of microcomputers in user areas, classrooms, and office space also will affect the temperature of the area. Photocopiers also generate an immense quantity of heat and require additional ventilation if they are located in an enclosed room that helps control noise as well.

Many other areas within a library generate noise. A large area with public access workstations and printers may be best located it in its own room or in an area well away from quiet study space. Strategies for deadening noise include good carpeting, the elimination of hard surfaces, and use of acoustic ceilings [58]. Multiple solutions will be needed throughout the building.

As with wiring, a flexible lighting plan will support future changes in the facility. The design should provide good general lighting throughout the library and apply special solutions as necessary [59]. In stack areas, for example, the positioning of the lighting is as important as the quantity of light reaching the lowest shelves. In most libraries, stack lighting is ceiling mounted, which makes it difficult, if not impossible, to change. Mudgett recommends stack-mounted lighting instead [60]. In areas where there are workstations either for the public or the staff, indirect or low lighting supplemented with task lighting may work well [61]. Decisions about task lighting for separate reading tables should be based on the individual situation. Within teaching or multimedia viewing rooms, the overall fluorescent lighting should be complemented by overhead incandescent lights controlled by a rheostat [62].

Metcalf writes extensively on the subject of stairs and elevators, or "vertical communication" [63]. In addition to the practical need for stairs, they also can serve as an aesthetic design element in the building. From the users' perspective, stairs and elevators should be easy to locate and should not cause disorientation when used. From a staff perspective, separate, staff-only, freight-quality elevators may be imperative. Federal, state, and local codes govern the placement and operation of stairs and elevators in public buildings.

Members of the building design review team should include representatives from the institution's security, fire, and/or environmental safety units. These representatives are familiar with code requirements and with institutional experiences that may or may not have been successful. Security for materials, equipment, and people within the library should be assured, as discussed by Metcalf [64]. Selection of a theft detection system must be compatible with the library's security needs, materials, and budget. Power needs and location should be reviewed, particularly proximity to metal or other equipment that may cause the system to malfunction. Nonpublic areas should be controlled with key, keypad, or card access systems that restrict access to authorized personnel. When planning a large building, locating staff on every floor assures the public of staff assistance. It is important to plan good sight lines from service points and to provide windows in the doors and walls of enclosed rooms. For after hours, motion detection systems may be considered.

Fire safety necessitates appropriate signage indicating emergency exits. Standards and codes for fire safety limit the occupancy of rooms, set the number of exits, dictate the types of construction materials that need to be used as firewalls or firebreaks in different areas, and specify the length of stair runs. With the demise of halon gas as a fire suppression system, sprinkler systems have become the fire control strategy of choice, supplemented by smoke detection. It is important to discuss with the architectural team the different sprinkler head options. Preaction sprinkler heads allow water to enter the system only when smoke is detected and release water only when the sprinkler head is heat activated. These specialized sprinkler head options may be more expensive and might only be used in special areas.

INTERIOR DESIGN CONSIDERATIONS

Many elements within the interior of the building have an impact on the services, flexibility, and longevity of the facility. The architect uses windows, window treatments, floor coverings, walls and ceilings, and light fixtures to enhance design, such as determining the shape of windows and the amount of natural light that enters the building. Wall colors and wall and floor coverings introduce color palates and textures that can be carried through the building. Wood imparts more warmth than brick, stone, or concrete. Ceiling, carpeting, and wall elements can direct the eye and the user to key areas of the building, a sort of subliminal guidance system. Light fixtures also provide ambience and direction. Many of these features facilitate and encourage the interaction between the building and its occupants.

Whether the interior designer is a separate consultant or from the architect's firm, it is important that all parties understand how the building is to feel or what impression the building should make. The building may have a different tone from area to area within the facility, from traditional to high-tech. The furnishings serve as another important interior design element. Some furniture may be custom-designed pieces; others may be purchased from catalogs. An inventory of current furniture helps determine what will be reused or replaced. Note that an inventory is extremely time-consuming and may, therefore, be best done by someone other than library staff.

The interior designer recommends the types of furnishings envisioned for the facility. The client usually has final approval concerning the proposed furnishings, including styles and colors. Insist on having people of varying sizes try out furniture, especially seating, whenever possible. If a piece of furniture, such as a study carrel, is being specially designed, the architect may build a prototype for evaluation. Ergonomic considerations include adjustable seating with lumbar support for computing space, lowered and adjustable keyboard trays, and footrests to relieve strain on the lower back. Classrooms may present another design challenge depending on the number of seats, equipment, layout, projection capabilities, and type of instruction envisioned [65].

Space and furnishings are even more crucial for the staff who live and work in the building all day. Provide natural light when possible. Encourage the staff to think about their workspace, including how the work flows, proximity to resources and each other, what they want their desktop to be like. Many technological infrastructure elements come into play here and should be kept in mind. Open-landscape, modular furniture has become increasingly popular because of its flexibility and the innovative ways storage and wire management can be handled [66].

Historical collections, meeting rooms, or lounge areas may require custom-designed furniture. It is very rare for a new facility to get all new furnishings, meaning that some furnishings from the current facility may have to be refinished or reupholstered. As a final recommendation when purchasing furnishings, buy the best quality possible within the budgetary limitations.

THE HOMESTRETCH

Eventually, the facility will be ready for occupancy. Metcalf provides a good overview concerning completion of construction, moving in, and occupying the facility [67]. The last months before building completion consume inordinate amounts of time and energy as walk-throughs take place, checklists are reviewed, furnishings arrive, and final installations occur. Staff benefit from detailed tours of the library, and they should engage in discussions to reexamine policies and procedures in light of the new facility. All the new features and systems must be tested. Telephones must be installed. The building needs to be thoroughly cleaned. Signage will be put into place, including room numbering. Unfortunately, not all these tasks will be done on time or concurrently. Most delays occur due to the late arrival of equipment and furnishings rather than delays in the completion of construction.

It may be possible to move part of the staff into the building as different sections are completed, but this creates security and operations complications. We highly recommend hiring a professional library-moving firm. Contact other libraries that have recently moved to see their scope of work and ask for advice. Expenses for a moving firm are rarely part of a construction budget. Mount's planning guide contains a detailed chapter that discusses moving the library [68]. After the move staff and users get comfortable with the new facility. This shakedown period varies in length as systems are fine-tuned and work continues with the architect, suppliers, and manufacturers. Plan on giving frequent tours and orientations of the facility, and be patient with those inevitable dissatisfied persons.

The final building dedication is best scheduled after a reasonable period of occupancy to allow for the full operation and furnishing of the building. This time of celebration may extend over a few days or even a week with special events connected to it. Appropriate acknowledgments should be given to everyone who has had a hand in the completion of the building, from the contractors and architects to the donors. The dedication must reflect the context of the institution and its traditions and customs. With good planning and careful attention to the myriad details of the building project, the institution will be proud of its successful new facility for many years.

REFERENCES

1. Shera J. Sociological foundations of librarianship. New York: Asia Publishing House, 1970:30.
2. Metcalf KD. Planning academic and research library buildings. 2nd ed. by Leighton PD and Weber DC. Chicago: American Library Association, 1986.
3. Hitt S. Administration: space planning for health sciences libraries. In: Darling L, Colaianni LA, Bishop D, eds. Handbook of medical library practice. 4th ed. v. 3. Chicago: Medical Library Association, 1988:387-466.
4. Twain M. The reports of my death are greatly exaggerated. In: Bartlett J. Familiar quotations. 13th ed. Boston: Little, Brown, 1955:679a.
5. Metcalf, op. cit., 590.
6. Snyder C. The building program statement (revisited). In: Martin RG. Libraries for the future: planning buildings that work. Chicago: American Library Association, 1992:41.
7. Lee H. Fundraising for the 1990's. Canfield, OH: Genaway, 1992.
8. Steele V. Becoming a fundraiser: the principles and practice of library development. Chicago: American Library Association, 1992.
9. Metcalf, op. cit., 57.
10. Ibid., 56-61.
11. Hitt, op. cit., 396.
12. Somerville AN. Planning: a cooperative effort. In: Mount E. Creative planning of special library facilities. New York: Haworth Press, 1988:53-64.
13. Hitt, op. cit., 396.
14. Brawner L. The roles of the building consultant and the planning team: part II. In: Martin RG. Libraries for the future: planning buildings that work. Chicago: American Library Association, 1992:35-37.
15. Hitt, op. cit., 397.
16. Metcalf, op. cit., 77-81.
17. Ibid., 62.
18. Ibid., 68.
19. Ibid., 68.
20. Thrun RR. The role of the architect in library planning. In: Mount E. Creative planning in special library facilities. New York: Haworth Press, 1988:67-71.
21. Michaels DL. Charette: design in a nutshell. Libr Adm Manage 1994;8(3):135-8.
22. Ibid., 135.
23. Ibid., 137.
24. Habich EC. Effective and efficient library space planning and design. In: McCabe GB, ed. Operations handbook for the small academic library. New York: Greenwood Press, 1989:301.
25. Ibid., 302.

26. Ibid., 303.

27. Hitt, op. cit., 402.

28. Metcalf, op cit., 29.

29. Ibid., 158.

30. Johnson J. Using space inventories, projections, and standards to build a successful program statement. In: Martin RG. Libraries for the future: planning buildings that work. Chicago: American Library Association, 1992:46.

31. Metcalf, op. cit., 151-58.

32. Fraley RA, Anderson CL. Library space planning. New York: Neal-Schuman, 1990:39-51.

33. Hitt, op. cit., 108-9.

34. University of Maryland, Baltimore. Capital improvement project facility program for the health sciences library: a new building for information services including the health sciences library. Baltimore, MD: UMBC rev. December 1991:33-35.

35. Metcalf, op. cit., 153.

36. Hitt, op. cit., 408.

37. Metcalf, op. cit., 157.

38. Hitt, op. cit., 409.

39. Ibid., 414.

40. Ibid., 419.

41. Metcalf, op. cit., 164-69.

42. Fraley, op. cit., 54-55.

43. Peters PE. Is the library a "place" in the age of networks? EDUCOM Rev 1994 Jan/Feb;29(1):62-3.

44. Association of College and Research Libraries. Standards for college libraries. 1995 ed. Available from Internet: http://www.acrl.org/acrl/guides/college.html.

45. Henshaw R. The library as a place: guest editorial. Coll Res Libr 1994 July;55(4):285.

46. Hitt, op. cit., 440.

47. Ibid., 425.

48. Johnson, op. cit., 48.

49. Marks, op. cit., 131.

50. Metcalf, op. cit., 242.

51. Hitt, op. cit., 139-141.

52. Metcalf, op. cit., 232.

53. Novak G. The forgiving building. Lib Hi Tech 1987 Winter; Consecutive Issue 20, 5(4):77-99.

54. Marks, op. cit., 129.

55. Ibid., 129.

56. Fisher T. Impact of computer technology on library expansions. Lib Adm Manage 1995 Winter;9(1):31-6.

57. Edwards HM. Planning for new technology. In: Edwards HM, ed. University library building planning. Metuchen, NJ: Scarecrow Press, 1990:102-8.

58. Novak, op. cit., 91.

59. Ibid., 81.

60. Mudgett JC. The role of the interior designer in library planning. In: Mount E. Creative planning of special library facilities. New York: Haworth Press, 1988:99-109.

61. Novak, op. cit., 84.

62. Ibid., 84.

63. Metcalf, op. cit., 149.

64. Ibid., 110-15.

65. Schulte L. Furnishing the electronic library. In: Mount E. Creative planning of special library facilities. New York: Haworth Press, 1988:111-31.

66. Ibid., 126.

67. Metcalf, op. cit., 505-25.

68. Mount E. Creative planning of special library facilities. New York: Haworth Press, 1988:35-40.

7

The Application of Systematic Research

Prudence W. Dalrymple

Research is systematic inquiry into a problem with the goal of gathering evidence to produce new knowledge [1].

The purpose of this chapter is to indicate how research on health information practice can contribute to optimal management in the health science information arena. Its central thesis argues that the systematic investigation of the problems encountered by health information professionals can contribute to improvements in how information professionals practice their profession. Participating in this enterprise either by directly engaging in research or by creating a work environment that supports the research activities of library staff is an important responsibility of library administrators. While researchable questions are by no means limited to the administrative realm, library managers hold the responsibility for the allocation of resources to investigate and address these issues. Thus, it is particularly appropriate for this discussion to appear alongside other management and administrative topics.

THE IMPORTANCE OF RESEARCH

Librarians and information professionals are realizing that the application of research methodologies plays a necessary part of professional practice. The research policy statement adopted by the Medical Library Association (MLA) in 1995 acknowledges the health sciences librarian's twofold relationship to research:

As managers of scientific knowledge, health sciences librarians play a key role in helping health care professionals to find scientific evidence that is applicable to individual practice decisions or to the complex task of developing clinical practice guidelines. As part of the health care enterprise, librarians must develop their own evidence-based information practice, identifying the methods and technologies that will provide the most cost-effective and high quality service in different health care, education, and research contexts [2].

Many other library and information science (LIS) associations advocate for the importance of developing a research base. Some have developed research agendas identifying topics of special interest or importance, although only a few have dedicated resources to supporting research activities. The overall output of library research was assessed a decade ago with "guarded optimism" [3].

The power of systematic investigation can be harnessed to enable practicing professionals to predict with more certainty the result of particular actions, understand certain behaviors or events, interpret and apply previous knowledge for problem-solving, or monitor progress toward the accomplishment of goals. Familiarity with the array of investigative and evaluative techniques enables the manager not only to confront problems with confidence but also to establish and solidify the place of the health information professional and the library or information center within the parent institution or user community.

The growing importance of information management in the delivery of health care requires that scientific inquiry be brought to bear on these problems. The niche that health sciences librarians occupy in contemporary society requires that they be able to select, evaluate, and interpret research reports both in their own field and in others. They also must be capable of conducting research, either as a member of a research team or by themselves. While health sciences librarians recognize that the investigation and solution of clinical health problems is an important goal for society, they have frequently limited their participation in the scientific enterprise to identifying and retrieving the cumulative knowledge of others as captured in the literature of the health sciences, rather than contributing to the creation of knowledge in the health information sciences. The development of practice guidelines based on scientific evidence for the wise deployment of library and information resources constitutes responsible librarianship, just as the development of clinical guidelines is crucial to responsible and effective health care.

Learning about research design and the use of research tools, such as statistics, is best done in the classroom or in guided study of the numerous excellent texts available. The reader seeking guidance in selecting reading materials may consult the research bibliography maintained and distributed through MLA's Library Research Section. MLA and other associations also offer numerous continuing education opportunities at professional meetings. Of particular interest to the health sciences librarian may be those courses aimed at evaluating and using the research literatures in library and information science and in medicine and allied health. Comprehensive, formal training in research methods can be obtained through college and university coursework, supplemented by formal continuing professional activities. Research skills may be applied and improved by investigating day to day library operations.

THE NATURE OF RESEARCH

Research, or systematic investigation, may be undertaken to enable results of policy and programmatic changes to be predicted and controlled, but often it is conducted simply to improve understanding of a phenomenon. Any professional who wants to interpret and apply effectively the findings of others to solve problems or increase understanding of current situations should possess a knowledge of research methodology. Applying the findings of research by being able to extract key information avoids "reinventing the wheel" or repeating past mistakes when confronted with a problem or difficult situation. Understanding the limits of knowledge prevents the manager from jumping to unwarranted conclusions. Administrators are frequently faced with operational and programmatic problems that must be resolved efficiently and effectively using a minimum of resources. They cannot afford to repeat mistakes, or they may need help in assessing the outcome of a new and untried approach.

Descriptions of the steps in research using the scientific method may vary slightly from textbook to textbook, but in general, scientific research consists of these steps:

1. State the problem in the form of a question.
2. Determine what, if anything, is known about the problem.
3. Design a methodology to investigate the question.
4. Gather and analyze data.
5. Report the results so that they may be incorporated into subsequent research.

Often, research is undertaken for evaluative purposes. While some scientists do not regard evaluation as true research, this chapter includes it because of its importance in library management. The evaluation of libraries and information systems and services is essential due to increasing competition for scarce resources and the requirement to demonstrate the impact of libraries on organizational effectiveness, corporate competitiveness, or patient outcomes.

Evaluation studies can demonstrate accountability to both funders and consumers. They can also be used to compare performance either against established norms or against targets established for internal purposes. Evaluative research allows health information professionals to develop "best practices," differentiate one course of action from another, and select a solution that is optimal for one's own particular situation.

The steps employed in evaluative research are based on those of the scientific method, but they are more pragmatic: question, learn, plan, observe, analyze, and report. Evaluative research assesses a phenomenon in terms of other similar phenomena, or in terms of typical or normative expectations. The goal of evaluation is not necessarily to create new knowledge but to evaluate one thing in terms of another.

The management and interpretation of the cumulated body of scientific knowledge are important aspects of health information practice. An understanding of research assists health information professionals, particularly those with administrative responsibilities, as they investigate problems, assess the research findings of others, and contribute to the scientific investigations of their colleagues.

TYPES OF RESEARCH

Research is often described in terms of the methods employed in the study, which generally fall into one of two categories: quantitative or qualitative. For many people, the term *research* denotes quantitative research using the scientific method. Qualitative and quantitative methods are both scientifically valid, and they can be used in complementary ways, even in the same investigation. Discussions that pit one methodology against the other can be misleading and may suggest a false dichotomy [4].

Quantitative Research

Quantitative research is so named because the *variables* are usually defined in such a way that they can be assigned a value and analyzed using statistical tests. Variables familiar to librarians include, for example, size of budget and size of collection. Understanding variables is critical because it affects the type of statistical tests that may be used for analysis. *Descriptive statistics* such as mean ("average"), mode ("typical"), and median ("midpoint") are familiar to most readers and appear frequently, even in newspapers and popular magazines. Quantitative research that uses *inferential statistics*, however, depends on random sampling and probability. A small sample, drawn correctly, can be assumed to represent a larger universe so that results can be generalized ("inferred") from the sample to the whole population. The accuracy with which this inference can be made is known as *probability*. Without at least a working knowledge of these ideas and a willingness to accept the conditions under which they operate, the reader of scientific research will be at a disadvantage. A very brief explanation of these concepts is included in the next section, but several of the references [5-7] may also prove useful.

Readers intending to undertake a research project, even though they may have had previous experience or education in research methods and statistics, are advised to review the appropriate sections in some standardized texts before developing a research design. Most experienced researchers have a favorite text or two, and if one presentation of a topic or statistical test is not clear, often another explanation will facilitate understanding. MLA's research bibliography, mentioned earlier, is a convenient way to keep abreast of new texts, and new works are reviewed in the LIS literature regularly.

Survey research is a common example of the use of sampling and statistical analysis to study a phenomenon. In survey research, *prediction* refers to forecasting what the results would be if the whole population were surveyed, rather than relying on a representative sample. When the sample is drawn correctly, sampling is actually preferable to surveying an entire population because it conserves resources, both human and fiscal, and assures the reliability and validity of the findings. Sampling is good discipline for the researcher because it forces stating the problem and defining the relevant variables carefully and precisely. A particularly good discussion of the statistical analysis of variables and scientific research may be found in the classic book by Kerlinger [8].

Selecting statistical tests that are appropriate to the variables under investigation is best done in consultation with someone knowledgeable in the area of statistical analysis. Often such individuals can be identified through a local college or university. Quite simply, statistical tests compare one situation to another to determine whether changes can be attributed to chance. Results are therefore reported in terms of the probability that the outcome was due to chance. The results of statistical tests are reported as being at the .0X level of significance. For example, it may be reported that there is a 5% or less likelihood that the results of a particular experiment were due to chance. This is reported as "statistically significant at the .05 level."

Results that are only 5% attributable to chance are far more meaningful than results that are 50% attributed to chance. Even better are results that are only 1% due to chance (significant at the .01 level). That is, it is much more desirable to predict the weather correctly 95% or 99% of the time, rather than only 50% of the time. A significance level of .01 means that in 99 of 100 cases where the exact same conditions are found, the results will be the same as those found under the experimental conditions. From this description, it is easy to see that quantitative research in the scientific tradition is ideally suited for predicting phenomena or establishing causality. A familiarity with the key concepts of random sampling and probability is essential in understanding quantitative research.

Qualitative Research

The conduct of qualitative research differs in several significant ways from quantitative research. The design usually focuses on a small sample, often employing a case study method. Data are collected through interviews and observation. For example, the National Library of Medicine (NLM) used the *critical incident technique*, a qualitative research approach, when it interviewed physician users of the MEDLINE system [9]. Qualitative studies frequently yield very large amounts of data, most of it narrative and verbal rather than numeric. Observations over an extended period of time can improve the credibility of the study because the researcher has adequate time in which to observe recurrent patterns of behavior. Data analysis may employ content analysis and descriptions that are continually refined and focused in an iterative process until patterns begin to emerge [10].

The value of qualitative research depends on the skill and knowledge of the researcher, who must be trained to be particularly sensitive to ways in which he or she may affect the outcome of the study, through subjective bias, intrusion into the environment, or unintentional selective observation. To avoid unintentional bias, the researcher also may apply principles of random sampling when selecting subjects to interview. Qualitative research, like quantitative research, still must be subjected to the scrutiny of the scientific community. The skill of the qualitative researcher may be revealed in the ability to identify and describe patterns and factors hitherto unnoticed. A brief introductory guide to qualitative research appears as part of a review article by Fidel [11].

Sometimes data patterns are more easily recognizable when a theoretical model guides them. Theory can be built from the top down or from the bottom up. *Top-down,* or *deductive,* theory may describe a situation in which a particular state of affairs is proposed and described because it seems logical or makes sense based on what is already known. The theory can then be tested using other research methods. This approach is also called *hypothesis testing* because the explanatory theory or hypothesis is tested through scientific investigation. In contrast, a *bottom-up,* or *inductive,* theory may be proposed after several investigations have been undertaken. In this case, theory emerges from the research findings themselves, rather than guiding the design of the research from the beginning. This approach also is referred to as *grounded* or *emergent theory.* Because both the data and the emergent theory are acknowledged to be situation-specific, it is difficult to generalize, but certain patterns may be identified in the data after a number of similar studies have been completed. These understandings may be transferred to other similar situations. When applying a theoretical model generated in one situation and applying it to another, the qualitative researcher must determine the comparability of the two situations, since random sampling and statistical analysis are generally not used.

OBJECTIVES OF RESEARCH

The most fundamental reason to undertake research is to answer a question. The degree to which a particular question can be answered may differ from field to field or from question to question. Researchers in the basic sciences aim to establish causality, to predict and control, while researchers in the social sciences may seek to improve their understanding of human behavior. For centuries scientific investigation has had the goals of creating new knowledge and establishing causality, contributing to a more understandable and predictable world. For example, basic medical research establishes the cause and treatment of disease. By studying genetic structures or patterns of viral contamination, the biomedical researcher investigates the origins of disease while clinical trials of therapeutic regimens are conducted to establish their effectiveness in controlling or eliminating pathology.

The scientific researcher uses the steps of the scientific method, beginning with a question or problem. To achieve the first goal—creating new knowledge—the researcher or scientist must next become familiar with what is known about the subject already. This is usually accomplished through a literature search to identify, acknowledge, and give credit to previous findings and then to build upon them. The phrase attributed to Sir Isaac Newton, "If I have seen further than others, it is by standing upon the shoulders of giants [12]," is a vivid way of emphasizing the importance of building on the cumulated knowledge in a field of inquiry. This knowledge provides guidance in what we might expect as a result of further scientific inquiry. Knowledge is expressed in a theoretical framework that explains a particular phenomenon.

When researchers seek to establish causality, they aim to demonstrate that B can be counted on to occur at each and every instance of A; that is, research and analysis must demonstrate the *reliability* of the finding. A statistical test can indicate that B will happen as a result of A at least 95% of the time (at the .05 level of significance). The research findings must also demonstrate that the laboratory result represents what happens in real life. The comparability between the laboratory findings and the actual phenomenon is called *validity*. Clearly, validity is a more difficult issue, particularly in behavioral research, such as psychology.

Many of the problems that health information professionals encounter have to do with human behavior, and research into these problems draws on the fields of sociology, psychology, and education, to name just a few. The problems faced by researchers in these areas do not lend themselves easily to prediction and control. This is partly because so many factors intervene that may affect outcomes but also because it is often impossible to conduct the necessary experiments to establish causality in human behavior. Nevertheless, systematic investigation of behavioral problems contributes to understanding and managing them. It can also determine the likelihood that one event will take place after another, thereby establishing patterns that facilitate systematic, advance planning for effective administration of library services.

THEORETICAL MODELS

Frequently, theoretical models guide the researcher in an investigation. Theories emerge from the cumulated knowledge about a particular phenomenon; a theory explains a phenomenon. When a scientist proposes a theory, the next step is to subject it to empirical testing. In its purest form, this kind of research is called *hypothesis testing* and may be described this way: If A, then B. The hypothesis is the statement "if A." To test this hypothesis, researchers design a study to determine whether B does indeed follow from each and every instance of A. For example, a librarian researcher may hypothesize that a decrease in the number of journals purchased will result in an increase in the number of interlibrary loan requests. To test this hypothesis, the librarian designs a study. Scientists submit their findings to the scrutiny of other researchers through the peer review and publication process. Publication not only disseminates the findings so that they can be applied, but it also makes the research available to others who may wish to test the theory further by changing the conditions slightly or by operationalizing the variables differently.

Theories are built on a set of assumptions about the world. Based on these assumptions, researchers develop theories that include propositional statements and hypotheses that can be tested. Sometimes these theories are so well integrated into our thinking that we scarcely recognize that they are based on a set of assumptions that may or may not be true or verifiable. For example, Darwin's theory of evolution explains the origin of the vast variety found among living organisms. Part of this theory is the notion of natural selection, or "survival of the fittest." While most biologists accept Darwin's theory because it explains natural phenomena, the application to sociology is less clear. Social Darwinism is both less testable because such experimentation could require creating situations that we would find ethically unacceptable but also because it does not explain social phenomena as neatly as the theory explains events in the natural world.

The theoretical assumptions or underpinnings of research must be taken into consideration when applying the results of research. Research findings should be examined with regard to both reliability (Do repeated measures yield consistent results?) and validity (Do the variables measure what they are assumed to measure?). For example, applying and using the results of research in educational testing can be problematic. The Scholastic Aptitude Test (SAT) is widely regarded as reliable because it yields similar results whenever it is administered to a sample population, but some question its validity. What does the SAT really measure? Does it predict academic performance only within the confines of narrowly defined educational system? If so, and if its limitations are acknowledged, it may still be useful. If, however, it is used as a surrogate for intelligence or as a predictor of success in life, it may be not only unreliable but also invalid.

Health information professionals and administrators must be familiar with a variety of research approaches and their reliance on assumptions so that they will not be limited in their ability to select appropriate methods and can use and interpret the findings of others intelligently. As two contemporary researchers note, there is a relationship

> between the assumptions of a methodology and the results that the methodology produces. . . . [T]he debate between qualitative and quantitative paradigms has helped to clarify that methodological issues and techniques represent not only constraints but also choices in the process of research [13].

The fundamental assumptions or worldview held by a researcher may well affect the approach selected to study the problem. Indeed, the worldview may even affect the selection of the problem itself.

While it is essential for the individual researcher to be aware of these often invisible and subtle biases, the administrator must also recognize that not everyone on the staff of the institution or the unit may approach problem solving in the same way. For this reason, administrators should state problems clearly and define variables and their measures carefully. Each step in the research design contributes to the outcome of the project and deserves attention if the results are to be understandable and useful to the organization. Even the choice of terminology carries with it a host of various meanings that can bias an investigation. For example, Dervin and Nilan review the various approaches to understanding the ubiquitous term *information* [14].

The rich results that can be obtained from using both a quantitative, positivist approach and a qualitative, interpretive one are described by Wildemuth [15]. She makes the point that the two approaches may be combined in ways that are well suited to provide comprehensive insight into the problem under investigation. While the nature of the research problem, rather than the personal philosophy of the researcher, is the criterion by which a research approach should be selected, individual researchers may be inherently more sympathetic to one approach or another, depending on their personal philosophy. They should nonetheless be alert to potential bias in both the design and conduct of the project regardless of the overall approach.

EVALUATIVE RESEARCH

When the first evaluative studies of library service were published, some librarians found the results shocking. The realization that a user may have a

60% chance of finding an item available in a library or less than a 60% chance of having a factual question answered completely and correctly prompted many library and information professionals to conduct additional studies and seek possible explanations for what seemed to be dismal performance [16-17]. The publication of these findings also raised questions about expectations for service and showed that little performance data about libraries was being used to improve service, or indeed, even to reflect performance norms. Ill-defined user expectations about libraries and library services and an absence of systematic evaluation within individual libraries and across groups of libraries have resulted in a lack of appropriate, meaningful, and realistic benchmarks against which performance can be measured. Fortunately, this situation is changing, for, as Lancaster observes, "evaluation is an essential element in the successful management of any enterprise" [18].

One approach to library evaluation that has become popular in recent years involves the use of output measures. In 1982, *Output Measures for Public Libraries* initiated a series of manuals aimed at various sectors of the library world [19-20]. It describes an approach through which an individual library sets its own goals and objectives for service, then measures its progress toward achieving these objectives. Output measures emerge from the context of a particular library and its environment and allow the administrator to evaluate performance in achieving goals and objectives. Despite their specificity, output measures provide a mechanism for systematically studying library services (outputs) and for defining variables that can be compared across similar communities. Defining or operationalizing variables is a first crucial step in scientific research and is the focus of the descriptive statistical studies that are described later in this chapter.

The health sciences library community has not adopted the output measures approach to the same extent as public libraries, but many libraries have been able to use research to demonstrate the impact of libraries on patient outcomes [21-23]. Little compares with the drama of life-and-death clinical situations; when scientific information is delivered to the bedside or surgical suite in time to save a patient's life, the critical role of the library enterprise is underscored. NLM was also instrumental in some of the early evaluations of information systems [24]. The effectiveness of information retrieval systems was one of the first areas of library and information science to undergo sustained research and evaluation. Lancaster's MEDLARS evaluation, along with the famous Cranfield studies, proposed two evaluative criteria for retrieval resulting from information systems: relevance and recall [25-27]. Dissatisfaction with the limitations of these measures spawned several decades of information retrieval research in which other measures were proposed. In fact, the information retrieval research literature is one of the best examples of basic research in the LIS field. The reader interested in reviewing this literature may wish to consult the *Annual Review of Information Science and*

Technology, an excellent source for becoming familiar with the overall production of basic research in information science.

Just as basic research must always answer the question "So what?" evaluative research must always engage the question "Compared to what?" Basic research establishes its value as it informs future research and contributes to theory building. On the other hand, evaluative research seeks to compare one situation to another and is not necessarily generalizable. The comparison may be within one institution, across time—yesterday compared to today—or it may be across institutions—my institution compared to yours, or mine compared to the average institution of similar type. When the findings from a group are similar, they can function as a de facto or empirical standard. Outcomes or impact research seeks to answer the "So what?" question by demonstrating that observable changes have occurred because of a particular series of events, personnel, or services. Demonstrating impact is not the same as establishing causality because it does not aim at prediction and control; rather, it aims to show the effect of a particular event.

ASSESSING THE RESEARCH RECORD

An important step in the research process, and one all too often overlooked, is the publication of results. In his book *Public Knowledge,* John Ziman provides an in-depth study of the nature of knowledge created from research endeavors and how society has a collective investment in the dissemination as well as the production of that knowledge [28]. Sharing the results of investigations has never been easier since electronic communication can make data and analysis available to scholars worldwide within seconds. Unfortunately, that development has also led to the publication of results prematurely and a proliferation of mediocre studies that place a burden on the reader to evaluate what is really worthwhile. For most of the twentieth century the peer review process provided a reliable gatekeeping function to ensure that the published literature reported only bona fide studies conducted according to accepted practice. Although the LIS literature has not yet been seriously affected by instances of scientific fraud, the community must not be complacent. In the LIS field, a greater problem may be the production and publication of flawed or insubstantial work [29].

While the dissemination of information is a common good, it places a burden on the consumer to discern what are useful and reliable results. As information professionals, librarians must take responsibility for the quality of the information they make available to their user community, whether in releasing the results of information searches or in selecting materials for the library collection. While intellectual access to information and freedom from censorship are fundamental values of the library profession, the health sciences librarian must also apply his or her evaluative skills in providing information services and resources to users. NLM identifies items that have been retracted, thus providing one kind of filter to the biomedical literature [30]. Unfortunately, most database producers have no such mechanism, and librarians searching for information in other disciplines must rely on their own analytical skills to recognize studies that are fraudulent or have been discredited. Understanding the research process and the paradigms in which research is carried out are essential skills for all information professionals.

APPLYING RESEARCH TO PRACTICE

Assessing research and applying findings can be facilitated when researchers clearly identify the variables of interest. The research should also make clear how these variables may change under various sets of circumstances. This is not always easy. The simple example of a book availability study serves to demonstrate how research may be used to improve and understand a problem in library management. The library manager may ask, "Why do users at Library X report more satisfaction finding books than at Library Y (my library)?" She may wonder, "What can be done to improve book availability?" The first step in finding an answer is to determine whether Library X and Library Y are truly comparable. If all the variables are defined clearly, one can determine, variable by variable, that the libraries are truly similar. Note that the libraries need not be the same in all ways, only in those that could be expected to affect the outcome. For example, the age of the library building may have no bearing on book availability while age of the collection might indeed have an effect on satisfaction. Next, the researcher defines and collects data on these variables that can then be used to compare the libraries based on the variables of interest.

Once differences or similarities in major variables of interest are established, the researcher can examine how a particular variable—the length of the loan period, for instance—affects book availability. A literature search for relevant research findings may reveal earlier testing of hypotheses on the effect of loan period on user satisfaction. Studies in which loan period is one of the defined variables may afford the manager some insight into its effect on user satisfaction. By isolating this variable (loan period), the researcher may demonstrate how book availability could be increased by manipulating the number of days a book circulates. The effect of loan period on volume of circulation transactions and staff workload must also be taken into consideration. The administrator will want to consider the trade-offs between an increased staff workload and user satisfaction when making a decision to change the services. The nature of the library environment (a busy clinical setting vs. an academic setting) may well affect the ultimate decision about the length of the loan period.

After reading the research literature and considering the library's environment, the manager may make an informed decision to change the length of the loan period based on the results of scientific investigation. She may also decide to collect data on user satisfaction and staff workload for a period of several months prior to making the change. This provides some baseline data against which to compare the research findings. Once the revised loan period has been in place for several months, the manager will once again collect some sample data on user satisfaction. After analyzing the data, the manager may report the findings to her staff or board, present them at a conference, and submit them for publication, thus contributing the research findings to the body of knowledge in library management.

In applying the findings of a research study, one must determine whether one's own situation is similar to or different from the one that is being described. Very few situations in life exactly replicate any other. Thus, it is important to know in which way a given problem resembles or differs from some other. Systematic investigation forces the clear articulation of each variable. Similarly, the various components of the situation change according to circumstances; for example, a library emphasizing journals differs from one in which the book collection overshadows the journals. Since libraries may differ substantially from one another, the ability to identify similarities and differences is essential to effectively applying research findings.

The information professional who wishes to examine qualitative approaches to a problem must demonstrate the applicability or relevance between the situation in which the research was conducted and the situation to which the findings are being applied. The structured nature of quantitative research, which includes clear definitions and operationalization of variables and the use of random sampling, can do much to assure the generalizability of the findings, yet the burden of demonstrating comparability between the situation described in a qualitative study and the research consumer's particular situation falls to the consumer. The qualitative researcher must take special care to describe the setting in full detail to assist the reader in assessing comparability. When the qualitative research employs abstractions that have evolved from a series of studies, the reader must further determine whether the authors have demonstrated adequately the connections between the abstractions and the data on which those abstractions are based [31].

An effective and healthy research community feeds back into the research process by replicating and testing research findings. An awareness of the collaborative nature of building a research base for practice is necessary if LIS is to build a sound foundation. Library managers frequently introduce new initiatives, often stimulated by problems that arise in practice or by developments that are introduced in the literature or at conference presentations. By approaching the proposed initiative as a field test, the library administrator can provide a substantive contribution to the LIS knowledge base while demonstrating the research process as part of the overall operations of the library. Field testing requires that there be a systematic and deliberate plan for introducing change. This plan should document preexisting conditions using quantitative measures if possible, predict outcomes based on stated assumptions, determine beforehand how and by what criteria and measures the change will be evaluated, ensure that appropriate observations are made throughout the process of change, adjust the variables to affect outcomes, and conclude with an evaluative analysis. Hewitt challenges the library administrator by stating:

> A sustained, cumulative, developmental/evaluative applied research effort, which uses replicable research designs and takes advantage of the almost limitless opportunities to conduct field research in a variety of settings, would no doubt have a profound impact on practice. . . . If such an effort is to be mounted, its required scale and the organization of the profession dictate that the library administrator play the key role in initiating and sustaining it [32].

Returning to the example of book availability, suppose that a library changed the length of its loan period in response to the findings presented earlier. This library, however, subsequently found that its results differed from those reported in the literature. After examining the situation carefully to compare it to what was reported, the librarian may suspect another variable is affecting the expected results. She may decide to write up the results of the library's experience, or she may decide to experiment further. This replication of the earlier study contributes to the body of cumulated knowledge and increases understanding. By identifying a new variable, the picture may at first seem more confusing, but by pursuing the investigation further, the situation may become clearer. Identifying variables and describing their interactions contributes to further understanding by providing a more sensitive and realistic model of the factors that affect a situation, in this case, book availability and user satisfaction. Collection size, loan period, and institutional setting may all affect one another. Each component of the model can be seen (and studied) in terms of the others. For example, user satisfaction could be the variable of personal interest, and it may be affected by loan period, collection size, institutional setting, and book availability.

Health sciences librarians practice in an environment that encourages applying research to practice. Faced with information overload, clinicians turn more and more to tools that manage the literature through critical review, assessment, and consolidation, and recently through meta-analysis. *Meta-analysis* is a technique that can be used to analyze and synthesize the results of a group of studies on a single topic. The combined results can then lead to development of practice guidelines.

The steps for meta-analysis are similar to those for standard scientific research:

1. State the problem.
2. Identify and select articles (data collection).
3. Extract data from articles.
4. Analyze data.
5. Present results [33].

The sheer volume of the clinical medical literature makes meta-analysis an attractive option for making scientific knowledge accessible to the practitioner. NLM has embarked on a program that facilitates the development of practice guidelines that may be based in part on meta-analysis. Librarians often contribute substantially to such projects because a thorough literature review is necessary to the appropriate conduct of a meta-analysis [34]. Meta-analysis appeals because of the obvious savings in time, effort, and resources and its potential to yield useful insights [35].

While a comparable volume of research and a similar degree of coordinated national leadership do not yet exist in library and information studies, distillation of research in a given area could do much to disseminate findings and potentially to lead to best practices for health sciences libraries. It should be noted that best practices or practice guidelines are based on research findings and are not simply "rules of thumb." If true practice guidelines are developed for health information professionals, such a development would represent an advance well beyond textbook management in that such guidelines would be grounded in scientific research that can be examined and tested.

CONTRIBUTING TO COLLABORATIVE RESEARCH

Libraries cooperate in a number of collaborative activities that enable individuals and groups to gain a better understanding of library practice and performance. Statistical data gathering and reporting is used by nearly all types of libraries to draw a picture of library performance in a particular domain [36]. Just as variables must be defined for research, variables must also be defined for gathering statistical data. The best statistical descriptions convey both understandable and useful messages. To achieve these objectives, researchers must define the variables carefully and design thoroughly the procedures for data collection. An accurate statistical profile depends on the participants' willingness and ability to contribute accurate and complete data. The quality of the data and the resulting profile improves if the subject is relevant to the participants in the study.

Such an activity requires that standardized measures be agreed on and that systematic and consistent approaches to data collection be employed. Staff must be trained in appropriate data-gathering processes, and internal quality control standards should be set. Otherwise, the results will be impressionistic at best and meaningless at worst. The Association of Research Libraries (ARL) and the Association of Academic Health Sciences Libraries (AAHSL) are two organizations that have undertaken the task of defining variables and coordinating cooperative data collection to facilitate comparisons across institutions and to improve understanding of their respective sectors of academic library practice. These aggregate data may be compared across a variety of institutions, using a large number of variables, or over a specified time period to discern trends, or both.

Collaboration among libraries has existed for a long time and has resulted in a number of innovative projects, a recent example of which is the twelve-library Internet collaborative known as HealthWeb [37]. Although such a project does not constitute research, it provides an interesting model for collaboration as well as a test bed for future evaluation. A more traditional approach to collaborative research is exemplified in the journal usage study conducted by thirty-six hospital libraries in cooperation with individual members of the Southern Chapter of the Medical Library Association. The results constitute a baseline of data that can be used in the future by this group and as a reference point for similar groups [38].

When the library compares its present performance to its past performance, it has full authority to define the variables on which it wishes to collect data, but, when national or regional norms are being established, the effort must be collaborative. Evaluation research, in particular, depends on the setting of benchmarks, either internal or external standards against which performance can be measured. Sometimes those standards are ideal models, but they are most meaningful if they are based on the real-world performance of actual libraries. To determine benchmarks, data must be collected across a number of libraries. These data are analyzed, and a comprehensive picture of performance is constructed. This complex and time-consuming process requires management skills as well as research expertise and institutional support and cooperation.

Internal performance standards often function as targets. These performance levels are meaningful in the context of the institution's own planning and evaluation process. Sharing the results of output evaluation can provide the basis for normative benchmarks, so long as they are developed with the same care as other statistical data.

Data gathering in libraries often centers on the use of surveys. Two common problems in library research include sending out a survey without pretesting it or distributing it in an uncontrolled fashion. Both errors consume the time and resources of librarians and users and will not yield meaningful results. Pretesting of survey instruments improves both reliability and validity. Making sure that respondents share a common understanding of the questions ensures that the answers will contribute to the researcher's overall framework for reporting the results of the survey. It also gives the researcher an idea of the range of likely responses so as to facilitate the analysis of the data. Although the library administrator may not be personally involved in all the data collection within the organization, the wise manager strongly encourages staff to follow accepted research practices and to strive for the highest-quality research possible, since it will inevitably reflect on the organization itself.

Sharing the results of surveys and, indeed, sharing the instruments themselves, can do much to streamline the research process. Creating a pool of pretested questions that can be incorporated into survey research could produce results more easily compared between or within institutions across time. At the very least, such questions would improve the quality of the surveys conducted by individual libraries.

Both the need and opportunity for interdisciplinary research in the LIS field has never been greater [39]. The changing nature of health information practice, the rapid growth of the Internet, and the rising need for providing consumers with accessible and credible health information present a full agenda of questions of interest to a large and diverse group of researchers. As a result, there are opportunities to form interdisciplinary research teams to investigate issues that arise from the impact of technology on libraries. Many problems that originally may have been of interest primarily to librarians have caught the attention of researchers from a variety of disciplines. The library administrator is often likely to be in the best position to identify, encourage, and facilitate possible partnerships that can strengthen the research base of health information practice.

CREATING AN ENVIRONMENT OF INQUIRY

The need for engaging in research extends beyond the academic community to clinical and corporate environments. A renewed emphasis on observing outcomes and establishing impact brought upon by the total quality management (TQM) and continuous quality improvement (CQI) movements suggest the widespread need for data-driven decision making in many institutions and organizations. Since very few information professionals practice outside an institutional framework, the degree to which institutions and their leaders support and reward research is critical to establishing a critical mass of research theory and findings.

While it can be argued whether the motivation necessary to conduct research comes from internal desire or external pressures (and thus whether the support for research should come from within or without), the point is that little harm can come from exerting administrative leadership in this area, and, quite probably, much positive benefit will accrue. Library administrators are in a position to act as catalysts, motivators, and supporters of investigative inquiry. A comprehensive list of institutional support factors appears in Dalrymple, Dahlen, and Stoddart; another list appears in Lee's article on library research committees [40-41]. Lee includes such practical suggestions as advising in the formulation of research proposals, reviewing proposals and recommending sources of support, offering editorial guidance, sponsoring research-related symposia, purchasing appropriate computer software and hardware, and publicizing opportunities for research and writing.

The final step of any research project is publishing the results in a peer-reviewed journal. Prior to submission, the authors can enlist colleagues in reading and critiquing the work, and they should be encouraged to do so in a way that is productive and helpful. The library administrator can do much to set a tone for staff to respond to each other's work in positive, collegial interactions. By modeling behavior in which initial drafts of work may be circulated for comment without fear of failure, criticism, or embarrassment, administrators (and others) can improve a work in progress, long before it is ready to be sent out for peer review. Indeed, research projects should be reviewed and critiqued throughout the duration of the project, and the responsibility of the library administrator includes providing that opportunity.

Basic responsibilities of the library administrator also encompass maintaining a professional reading collection available to staff, encouraging its use through routing and journal clubs, and facilitating document delivery. Librarian researchers should be provided the same level of access to the library's services and resources as general library users. Encouraging in-library discussions and reviews of research findings, particularly as they may apply to real-life problems, can encourage the use of research and develop understanding of how to interpret research findings. Such discussion creates an environment that values collaboration and cooperative approaches to problem solving. Few scientific discoveries are made in isolation, and most research projects are undertaken jointly. Shared ownership of library problems, along with a commitment to engage in their collaborative investigation and solution, leads to an environment supportive of research and investigation. In fact, it can be argued that effective research undergirds daily practice even when the practitioner does not recognize it.

MLA AND RESEARCH

Like many other associations, the Medical Library Association has increasingly recognized the role and importance of research. An important event in catalyzing the current emphasis on research was Erika Love's 1979 presidential address naming research as the third dimension of librarianship, after education and practice [42]. As MLA president, she appointed an Ad Hoc Committee to Study MLA's Role in Library Related Research; the activities of this group eventually resulted in the formation of the current Research Section. The section has undertaken a number of subsequent activities and has been instrumental in providing a forum for health sciences librarians to acknowledge collectively the importance of fostering research in the field. Carla Funk, MLA executive director, notes that the evolving nature of the *Bulletin of the Medical Library Association* "may be thought of as the fuel for achieving the Association's goals" [43]. As such, the journal's mission statement of "reporting research, development, and activities in the field of health sciences librarianship" describes its key role in fostering the exchange of information and knowledge gained from research. Recently, the scope of articles section of the *Bulletin's* "Information for Authors" was rewritten, stating that the *Bulletin* "aims to advance the practice and research knowledge base of health sciences librarianship" [44].

The 1995 MLA research policy statement lays out clearly the joint responsibility of educators, administrators, health care professionals, researchers, policymakers, and funders to establish an environment that is conducive to increased production and use of research [45]. The policy statement characterizes an environment that provides

- access to a broad range of relevant education and training,
- advice and assistance for librarians embarking on research,
- adequate research funding,
- incentives for collaborative research,
- flexible and supportive employment situations, and
- recognition for research work.

Through its vigorous emphasis on the vital role of research, funding of specific projects, and publication of key studies, MLA fosters a professional focus on basic and applied library research. It offers continuing education courses that enhance knowledge of research theory and skill in employing specific technologies described in this chapter. Yet, ultimately, research depends on individuals.

The library administrator clearly has a key role to play in advancing research that expands the work of the health information professional. Whether by conducting systematic inquiry into problems or questions of his or her own choosing or by supporting the inquiry of others, the library administrator both contributes to and benefits from research. Investment in research will improve library services and management over time; hence, it represents an administrative tool that cannot be overlooked.

REFERENCES

1. Medical Library Association. Using scientific evidence to improve information practice: the research policy statement of the Medical Library Association. Chicago: Medical Library Association, 1995.

2. Ibid., 4.

3. McClure CR, Bishop AP. The status of research in library/information science: guarded optimism. Coll Res Libr 1989 Mar;50(2):127-43.

4. Sandstrom AR, Sandstrom PE. The use and misuse of anthropological methods in library and information science research. Libr Q 1995 Apr;65(2):161-99.

5. Miller DC. Handbook of research design and social measurement. 4th ed. New York: Longman, 1983:1-68.

6. Hernon P, et al. Statistics for library decision-making. Norwood, NJ: Ablex, 1989.

7. Kerlinger FN. Foundations of behavioral research. 3rd ed. New York: Holt, Rinehart, Winston, 1986.

8. Ibid.

9. Lindberg DA, Siegel ER, Rapp BA, Wallingford KT, Wilson SR. Use of MEDLINE by physicians for clinical problem solving. JAMA 1993 Jun 23-30;269(2):3124-9.

10. Westbrook L. Qualitative research methods: a review of major stages, data analysis techniques, and quality controls. Libr Inf Sci Res 1994;16:243-9.

11. Fidel R. Qualitative methods in information retrieval research. Libr Inf Sci Res 1993;15:219-47. Also available from Internet: http://www.geocities.com/~spanovdi/quote.html.

12. Merton R. On the shoulders of giants: a Shandean postscript. Chicago: University of Chicago Press, 1993:vii.

13. Bradley J, Sutton B. Reframing the paradigm debate. Libr Q 1993 Oct;63(4):407.

14. Dervin B, Nilan M. Information needs and information uses. In: Williams M, ed. Annual Review of Information Science and Technology. White Plains, NY: Knowledge Industry, 1986:3-33.

15. Wildemuth B. Post-positivist research: two examples of methodological pluralism. Libr Q 1993 Oct;63(4):450-68.

16. Mansbridge J. Availability studies in libraries. Libr Inf Sci Res 986;8:299-314.

17. Crowley T, Childers T. Information services in public libraries: two studies. Metuchen, NJ: Scarecrow Press, 1971.

18. Lancaster WF. If you want to evaluate your library. London: Library Association, 1988.

19. Zweizig DL, Rodger EJ. Output measures for public libraries: a manual of standardized procedures. Chicago: American Library Association, 1982.

20. Van House NA, et al. Output measures for public libraries. 2nd ed. Chicago: American Library Association, 1987.

21. Marshall JG. Impact of the hospital library on clinical decision making: the Rochester study. Bull Med Libr Assoc 1992 Apr;80(2):169-78.

22. King DN. The contribution of hospital library information services on clinical care: a study in eight hospitals. Bull Med Libr Assoc 1987 Oct;75(4):291-301.

23. Klein MS, et al. Effect of online searching on length of stay and patient care costs. Acad Med 1994;69(6):489-95.

24. Lancaster FW. Evaluation of the MEDLARS demand search service. Bethesda, MD: National Library of Medicine, 1968.

25. Cleverdon CW. Report on testing and analysis of an investigation into the corporate efficiency of indexing systems. Cranfield, England: College of Aeronautics, 1962.

26. Cleverdon CW, Keen M. ASLIB Cranfield Research Project: factors determining the performance of smaller type indexing systems. v. 2. Bedford, England: Cleverdon, 1966.

27. Cleverdon CW, Mills J, Keen M. ASLIB Cranfield Research Project: factors determining the performance of smaller type indexing systems. v. 1. Bedford, England: Cleverdon, 1966.

28. Ziman J. Public knowledge: an essay concerning the social dimension of science. London: Cambridge University Press, 1968.

29. Hernon P, Altman E. Misconduct in academic research: its implications for the service quality provided by university libraries. J Acad Libr 1995 Jan;21(1):27-37.

30. Kotzin S, Schuyler PL. NLM's practices for handling errata and retractions. Bull Med Libr Assoc 1989 Oct;77(4):337-42.

31. Bradley J. Methodological issues and practices in qualitative research. Libr Q 1993 Oct;63(4):447.

32. Hewitt JA. The role of the library administrator in improving LIS research. In: McClure CR, Hernon P, eds. Library and information science research: perspectives and strategies for improvement. Norwood, NJ: Ablex, 1991:163-78.

33. McKibbon A, Walker-Dilks C. Panning for gold: how to apply research methodology to search for therapy, diagnosis, etiology and prognosis articles. Rochester, NY: Rochester Regional Library Council. Rochester General Hospital, 1994.

34. Mead TL, Richards DT. Librarian participation in meta-analysis projects. Bull Med Libr Assoc 1995 Oct;83(4):461-4.

35. Moher D, Olkin I. Meta-analysis of randomized controlled trials: a concern for standards. JAMA 1995 Dec 27;274(24):1962-4.

36. Fingerman J. Painting the picture: personal computers and graphical presentation of statistics. Libr Adm Manage 1989 (Fall);3:199-204.

37. Redman PM, Kelly JA, Albright ED, et al. Common ground: the HealthWeb project as a model for Internet collaboration. Bull Med Libr Assoc 1997 Oct;85(4):325-30.

38. Dee CR, Rankin JA, Burns CA. Using scientific evidence to improve hospital library services: Southern Chapter/Medical Library Association journal usage study. Bull Med Libr Assoc 1998 Jul;86(3):301-6.

39. Humphreys BL. Librarians and collaborative research: towards a better scientific basis for information practice. Bull Med Libr Assoc 1996 Jul;84(3):433-6.

40. Dalrymple PW, Dahlen KH, Stoddart J. Imperatives for continuing research education: results of a Medical Library Association survey. Bull Med Libr Assoc 1992 Jul;80(3):213-8.

41. Lee TP. The library research committee: it has the money and the time. J Acad Libr 1995 Mar;21(2):111-5.

42. Love E. Research: the third dimension of librarianship. Bull Med Libr Assoc 1980 Jan;68(1):1-5.

43. Funk CJ. In support of research. Bull Med Libr Assoc 1992 Oct;80(4):385.

44. Homan MJ. Revision of BMLA information for authors. Bull Med Libr Assoc 1999 Jan;87(1):93-4.

45. Medical Library Association, op. cit.

Appendix A

Compilation of Skills Recommended for Careers in Health Sciences Librarianship

Health Information Science Knowledge and Skills, from the Medical Library Association's *Platform for Change*

- *Health sciences environment and information policies:* understanding of the contexts in which the need for biomedical and related information emerges and the unique ways of perceiving and interpreting those environments
- *Management of information services:* leadership in the application of library and information science to the handling of health sciences information resources in complex institutional environments
- *Health sciences information services:* knowledge of the content of information resources and skills in using them; understanding of the principles and practices related to providing information to meet specific user needs and to ensure convenient access to information in all forms
- *Health sciences resource management:* knowledge of the theory and skills involved in identifying, collecting, evaluating, and organizing resources and developing and providing databases
- *Information systems and technology:* understanding and use of technology and systems to manage all forms of information
- *Instructional support systems:* ability to provide instruction in accessing, organizing, and using information to solve problems
- *Research, analysis, and interpretation:* responsibility to explore the fundamental nature of biomedical information storage, organization, utilization and application in learning, patient care, and the generation of new knowledge

Highly Ranked Skills from the Vanderbilt University Study

- Initiative
- Assertiveness
- Flexibility
- Proactivity
- Capacity for lifelong learning
- Marketing
- General librarianship
- Health sciences knowledge
- Medical informatics
- Technical skills
- Institutional and managerial knowledge
- Education
- Research
- Finances and fund-raising

Skills Ranked Most Important from the University of Pittsburgh Study

- Information systems/technology
- Information services
- Information retrieval
- Internet/database resources
- Telecommunications
- Health sciences information sources
- Database resources
- Oral/written communication

Professional Competencies Identified in *Professional and Personal Competencies for the Special Librarian of the 21st Century* from the Special Libraries Association (SLA)

- Has expert knowledge of the content of information resources, including the ability to evaluate and filter them critically
- Has specialized subject knowledge appropriate to the business of the organization or client
- Develops and manages convenient, accessible and cost-effective information services that are aligned with the strategic directions of the organization
- Provides excellent instruction and support for library and information service users
- Assesses information needs and designs and markets value-added information services and products to meet identified needs

- Uses appropriate information technology to acquire, organize, and disseminate information
- Uses appropriate business and management approaches to communicate the importance of information services to senior management
- Develops specialized information products for use inside or outside the organization or by individual clients
- Evaluates the outcomes of information use and conducts research related to the solution of information management problems
- Continually improves information services in response to changing needs
- Is an effective member of the senior management team and a consultant to the organization on information issues

Personal Competencies Identified by SLA

- Is committed to service excellence
- Seeks out challenges and sees new opportunities both inside and outside the library
- Sees the big picture
- Looks for partnerships and alliances
- Creates an environment of mutual respect and trust
- Has effective communication skills
- Works well with others in a team
- Provides leadership
- Plans, prioritizes, and focuses on what is critical
- Is committed to lifelong learning and personal career planning
- Has personal business skills and creates new opportunities
- Recognizes the value of professional networking and solidarity
- Is flexible and positive in a time of continuing change

Appendix B

Annotated Bibliography of Library Space Planning

Ball MJ, Weise FO, Freiburger GA, Douglas JV, eds. Building the library/information center of the future. Special Issue. Comp Methods Programs in Biomed 1994 Sept;44(3/4):141-270. The papers included in these proceedings range from descriptions of renovation projects to visions of the future, from an explanation of the changing medical curriculum to an in-depth view of a planning process. They provide some answers and serve as a guide to asking the right questions.

Bastille J. Planning library facilities. In: Bradley J, ed. Hospital library management. Chicago: Medical Library Association, 1983:266-93. This chapter provides useful guidance for library facilities in hospitals.

Bazillion RJ, Braun C. Libraries as high-tech gateways: a guide to design and space decisions. Chicago: American Library Association, 1995. This work describes how traditional library functions and electronic information services can be accommodated in the same building. Includes a chapter on the library as a "teaching instrument."

Brown CR. Selecting library furniture: a guide for librarians, designers, and architects. Phoenix: Oryx Press, 1989. This book guides decision makers through the selection process for freestanding furniture such as chairs, tables, shelving units, and more (carpets, floor coverings, lights, etc., are not covered). Brown discusses the process for determining furniture requirements and provides examples of applying the process to particular items. Background information about construction follows with discussion of particular kinds of furnishings and shelving available. The final chapters address the bid procedures and the library market. A bibliography and a list of manufacturers are included.

Cirillo SE, Danford RE. Library buildings, equipment and the ADA. Chicago: American Library Association, 1996. This book offers library-specific guidance for complying with ADA requirements.

Cooper W. Integrating information technologies for the library environment. Libr Adm Manage 1994;8(3):131-4. Cooper discusses the importance of the information technology infrastructure in the design or renovation of a library building.

Duncan JM. The information commons: a model for (physical) digital resource centers. Bull Med Lib Assoc 1998 Oct;86(4):576-82. This paper describes a facility, its programmatic elements, and its impact on education, communication, and technology in an academic health science setting. Includes floor plan with square feet, staffing requirements, and plans for expansion.

Edwards HM. Planning for new technology. In: University library building planning. Metuchen: Scarecrow Press, 1990:102-8. This chapter discusses new technology and its impact on planning the library of the future. It considers various environment and design problems relating to the computer room, such as security, power supply, and space requirements. A very complete checklist for computer installation developed by B. G. Toohill is provided.

Fisher T. Impact of computer technology on library expansions. Libr Adm Manage 1995 Winter;9(1):31-6. Although focusing on projects developed by the author's architectural firm, this article offers concrete suggestions and solutions for addressing technological concerns such as wiring, power, and the like.

Fraley RA, Anderson CL. Library space planning. New York: Neal-Schuman, 1990. An invaluable, practical guide for the library faced with moving, whether it be into a new building or a reorganization of current space. Fraley and Anderson explain in detail the steps involved in moving a collection, with suggestions for generating publicity, measuring the collection, estimating the time involved and the people needed, and determining how to keep the library running during the move. Many excellent diagrams and illustrations accompany the text. The appendix contains a sample bid document and a bibliography. This is one of the best sources for planning a move into the new building.

Habich EC. Effective and efficient library space planning and design. In: McCabe CB, ed. Operations handbook for the small academic library. New York: Greenwood Press, 1989:301-11. This chapter offers practical suggestions for the design of libraries that meet the criteria of "effective and efficient." Beyond defining those terms as they relate to libraries, the author suggests use of bubble diagrams to discover functional relationships. This chapter lays a good foundation for the planning process.

Hawthorne P, Martin RG, eds. Planning additions to academic library buildings: a seamless approach. Chicago: American Library Association, 1995. Case studies are presented from Hope College, Western Maryland College, and the University of Washington. Each presents very different problems and site issues to overcome. Floor plans are included. Appendix B offers a checklist of additions to academic library buildings with library contacts and architectural firms associated with the items.

Henshaw R. The library as a place: guest editorial. Coll Res Libr 1994 July;55(4):283-5. A concise response to questions concerning the need for new library buildings, based on an examination of future roles libraries will fill.

Hitt S. Administration: space planning for health science libraries. In: Darling L, Colaianni LA, Bishop D, eds. Handbook of medical library practice. 4th ed. v. 3. Chicago: Medical Library Association, 1988; 387-466. From the standard text for health sciences libraries, this chapter focuses on planning, constructing, and occupying a new library building.

Kaufman PT, Mitchel AH. 2001: A space reality: strategies for obtaining funding for new library space. SPEC Kit 200. Washington, DC: Association of Research

Libraries, 1994. Program statements from seven university libraries to justify requests for library space. Some include data, statements and requests from users, and predictions of what changes will take place in the future.

King HM. Academic library buildings for the next century: insights from the United States. LASIE 1998 Mar: 29(1):21-31. As part of the preliminary planning process for three library building projects at La Trobe University, the author studied fifteen new or recently remodeled academic library buildings in the United States. She examines electronic infrastructures and future-proofing strategies, new kinds of space and services, impacts on traditional space and services, effective distribution of space and services and new space norms, design trends symbolizing the library's changing role, colocation with compatible facilities, and the underlying philosophy of the academic library of the future that has driven the planning of the projects visited.

Kruhly JO. The new library on college and university campuses. Washington, DC: KPMG Peat Marwick, 1992. A report by KPMG Peat Marwick that enumerates current architectural issues to consider in renovating an existing library or building a new one from an architect's point of view.

Lee H-W, Hunt GA. Fundraising for the 1990's: the challenge ahead: a practical guide for library fundraising, from novice to expert. Canfield, OH: Genaway, 1992. The authors offer practical information for fundraising. Includes case studies and an entire chapter on the concept of stewardship.

Leighton PD, Weber DC. Planning academic and research library buildings. 3rd ed. Chicago: American Library Association, 1999, © 2000. The classic text on planning library buildings, originally written by Keyes Metcalf, covers all aspects of planning a new library building, from the beginning stages of planning through interior design, selection of the architect through moving into the new building. The appendices contain examples of programs to guide the librarian who is beginning to write a plan, equipment lists, formulas and tables for calculating seating and shelving, a bibliography, and a glossary.

Library Administration and Management Association. American Library Association. Planning library buildings: a select bibliography. Chicago: American Library Association, 1990. Both journals and books are covered. Most works cited were published since 1980. Author index. The bibliography is arranged by subject and covers topics such as planning, mechanical and structural systems, automation, interior design, financing, and moving. It also cites selected case studies.

Lucker J. Negotiating the rocky shoals: the politics of building a library. In: Is the library a place?: Minutes of the meeting of the Association of Research Libraries (118th, Quebec, May 15-17, 1991). Washington, DC: Association or Research Libraries, 1991. Whether building a new library or renovating an existing facility, a delicate balance is required to bring together all of the stakeholders (administrators, trustees, individual donors, staff, patrons and architects) who wish to influence the planning and design. Lucker creatively links the rules that govern library building to the rules and laws that govern nature and everyday life.

Marks KE. Planning for technology in libraries. N C Libr 1991 Fall;49:128-31. Marks see electronic technology as an indispensable element that must be fully integrated into the work and service of the library. Five areas demanding serious consideration are discussed: electrical power, conduits, lighting, furniture, and air temperature/quality.

Martin RG, ed. Libraries for the future: planning buildings that work. Chicago: American Library Association, 1992. The edited proceedings of a conference sponsored by the Buildings for College & Research Libraries Committee of ALA and cosponsored by the Architecture for Public Libraries Committee of ALA. Papers cover the roles of the consultant, the planning team, and outlines of the process. An excellent overview of the trends and issues confronting librarians approaching the building process, with strong emphasis on understanding the mission and purpose of the library, and the functional requirements of the library. The building program statement is covered in two papers. Functional and technical requirements are discussed in relation to building criteria and space relationships. Suggestions are given on choosing an architect and on the composition of the design team.

Matier M, Sidle CC. What size libraries for 2010? Plan Higher Ed 1993 Summer;21:9-15. Discusses the need for library space based on emerging technologies. Recommends planning space in conventional terms until the year 2000 but, after that, planning for more remote storage and technology to handle additional space needs.

Michaels DL. Charette: design in a nutshell. Libr Adm Manage 1994;8(3):135-8. Discusses the benefits of the charette as an architectural planning process to break down barriers among those involved.

Mount E. Creative planning of special library facilities. New York: Haworth Press, 1988. This book describes itself as "an introductory text for those who have had little or no experience in . . . designing a facility." It is intended primarily for smaller, more specialized libraries. All aspects of planning a library are covered including preplanning suggestions. Extensive, annotated bibliography and four libraries recently renovated or newly built each have a chapter.

Potter C. What do you do when the answer is yes? planning technology for a new academic library. Illinois Libr 1996 Summer;78:124-6. Description of goals, planning process, and technology requirements.

Rettig JR. Designing scenarios to design effective buildings. In: La Guardia C, ed. Recreating the academic library. New York: Neal-Schuman, 1998:67-89. The need for user-centered design is discussed as well as design for behavioral changes. The author encourages using scenario planning.

Rizzo J. Ten ways to look at a library. Am Libr 1992 Apr;23(4):322-6. Rizzo briefly discusses ten different roles a library can play and how architectural design should respond. The author advocates that in planning or renovating a library, librarians should look at the structure as users, trustees, staff, or planners might see it.

Sannwald WW, ed. Checklist of library building design considerations. Chicago: American Library Association, 1991. Questions on every aspect of space and function in a library are provided, including communications equipment, electrical requirements, and shelving. Each section has one or more questions relating to accessibility for users with disabilities. A very straightforward, easy-to-use approach to planning, covering specific needs (e.g., coat closets) and broad issues.

Steele V, Elder SD. Becoming a fundraiser: the principles and practice of library development. Chicago: American Library Association, 1992. This book discusses the challenge of maintaining traditional services while offering new technology-driven services. Clearly written, it addresses the issues and vagaries of fund-raising in addition to good, practical suggestions for pitfalls to avoid and strategies for success.

Trinkley M. Preservation concerns in construction and remodeling of libraries: planning for preservation. Columbia: Chicora Foundation, 1992. The goal of this publication is to help libraries incorporate preservation concerns in such building activities as new construction, renovations, and routine maintenance. The text provides a variety of techniques that allow preservation concerns to be integrated into site selection, the design of the building envelope, the library interior, floor coverings, selection of roofing materials, electrical wiring, and plumbing features.

Williams DE. Reengineering existing buildings to serve the academic community. In: Pitkin GM, ed. The national electronic library: a guide to the future for library managers. Westport, CT: Greenwood Press, 1996:85-97. This chapter discusses elements that must be considered in planning to rework or remodel existing buildings. Deals with special concerns such as electronic systems, lighting, power and telecommunications, walls, mechanical systems, noise, and furniture.

Glossary

AAHSL	Association of Academic Health Sciences Libraries (formerly Association of Academic Health Sciences Library Directors).
AAMC	Association of American Medical Colleges
ACRL	Association of College and Research Libraries (ALA)
Alliance	Colorado Alliance of Research Libraries
AMIA	American Medical Informatics Association
Ariel	Document transmission system (The Research Libraries Group, Inc.)
ARL	Association of Research Libraries
ARPA	Advanced Research Project Agency
ARPANET	Advanced Research Projects Agency Network
BACS	Bibliographic Access and Control System (Washington University, St. Louis)
BCG	Boston Consulting Group
BRS	Bibliographic Retrieval Services (online service now called CDP Online)
BVE	Bound volume equivalents
CCC	Copyright Clearance Center
CD-ROM	Compact disc, read-only memory
CINAHL	Cumulative Index to Nursing & Allied Health Literature
CNI	Coalition for Networked Information
CQI	Continuous quality improvement
DOCLINE	Documents Online (NLM)
DocView	Experimental document viewing system (NLM)
DOE	Department of Energy (U.S.)
EBP	Evidence-based practice
EEOC	Equal Employment Opportunity Commission
FOLUSA	Friends of Libraries U.S.A.
FTE	Full-time equivalent
GIR	Group on Information Resources (AAMC)
GPEP	General Professional Education of the Physician
Grateful Med	User-friendly software for searching the MEDLARS system (NLM)

206

Administration and Management

HEPNET	High Energy Physics Network
HII	Health Information Infrastructure
HPCC	High Performance Computer and Communication Act
IAIMS	Integrated Advanced Information Management Systems (was Integrated Academic Information Management Systems)
ICOLC	International Coalition of Library Consortia
ILL	Interlibrary loan
Internet	Network of networks using standard telecommunications protocol
IP	Internet protocol
IS	Information system
JCAHO	Joint Commission on Accreditation of Healthcare Organizations
JSTOR	Journal Storage project
LAMA	Library Administration and Management Association (ALA)
LC	Library of Congress
LIS	Library and information science
Loansome Doc	Document-ordering feature of the Grateful Med software (NLM)
MARC	Machine-readable cataloging
MEDLIB-L	Medical libraries discussion list on the Internet
MEDLINE	MEDLARS Online (database—NLM)
MFENet	Magnetic Fusion Energy Network
MIS	Medical Informatics Section (MLA)
NII	National Information Infrastructure
NLM	National Library of Medicine
NSF/Net	National Science Foundation Network
OCLC	Online Computer Library Center (Ohio)
Octanet	Automated interlibrary loan project (Midcontinental RML)
OhioLINK	Library consortium for information services, resource sharing, and document delivery (Ohio)
OPAC	Online public access catalog
OSHA	Occupational Safety and Health Act
OSU	Ohio State University
PACS-L	Public Access Computer Systems discussion list on the Internet
PBL	Problem-based learning
PCP	Primary care provider
PHILSOM	Periodical Holdings in Library of School of Medicine (Washington University, St. Louis)

QuickDOC	Program for offline data entry and ILL file maintenance in the DOCLINE system (Beth Israel Hospital)
QWL	Quality of work life
SAT	Scholastic Aptitude Test
TCP	Transmission control protocol
TQM	Total quality management
UCLA	University of California, Los Angeles
UCSB	University of California, Santa Barbara
UMBC	University of Maryland, Baltimore Campus
UMLS	Unified Medical Language System
UnCover	Document-ordering system (CARL Systems, Inc.)
WAIS	Wide area information service
WGU	Western Governors University
WWW	World Wide Web

Index

This is primarily a subject index. Personal authors of works cited in the text are not indexed. Acronyms and abbreviations are given preference as indexing terms if they are more commonly used than the full names of organizations or publications.

academic health sciences libraries:
    curriculum-based instruction in, 109;
        and health professional training, 4;
        and hospital mergers, 3; IAIMS'
        roles, 6; job descriptions from, 39;
        marketing scenario for, 95 (*see also*
        marketing); peer review in, 64;
        responsibility-centered
        management in, 22–23; student
        workers for, 43; survey of
        computer-systems in, 111
access services, 159
access *versus* ownership, 25–27, 135
advertising, 88
affirmative action, 46, 51
American Medical Informatics Association,
    118
American Society for Information Science,
    27
Americans with Disabilities Act, 1991, 48
*Annual Review of Information Science
    and Technology*, 182–83
architects, 140–41, 143–47
Ariel, 112–13
ARPANET, 104

Association of Academic Health Sciences
    Libraries, 50, 112, 124, 188
Association of Academic Health Sciences
    Library Directors, 111
Association of American Medical Colleges,
    109, 113, 119
Association of College and Research
    Libraries, 46, 58, 152–53, 155
Association of Research Libraries, 27, 29,
    58, 188
authoring software, 118

BACS, 106
benchmarks, determination of, 188
blueprints, architectural, 148
budgeting:
    for building, 137–38;
    calendar for, 21;
    and institutional policy, 21–23;
    and responsibility-centered
        management, 22–23;
    steps in, 20–21;
    and strategic planning, 20;
    for technological development, 127–28;
    types of budgets, 21–22

*Bulletin of the Medical Library
    Association*, 191
burnout, 66–67

capital expenses, 25
CARL UnCover, 113
carrels, study, 156, 168
CD-ROM technology, 108
Challenge to Action, 41, 54
chiropractic libraries, 41
circulation desks, 163–64
Civil Rights Act, 1964, 45, 63
Civil Rights Act, 1991, 45
classrooms, library, 157, 167–68
Coalition for Networked Information
    (CNI), 118
Cochrane Collaboration, 114
*Code of Ethics for Health Sciences
    Librarianship*, 103
collections, library, 151–54
collective bargaining, 46–47
compensation plans, 59–61
conference rooms, 161
consultants, 136, 141
consumer health information services, 3–4,
    79, 94, 121
contracting for services, 27–28
Copyright Clearance Center, 117
corporate partnerships, 32
cubook formula, 153

dental libraries, 41
digital library, 122
distance learning, 117, 157
DOCLINE, 107–8
document delivery, 108, 112–13, 160
DocView, 112–13
donors, library, 141–42

Electronic Collections Online (ECO), 119
electronic discussion lists, 112
electronic resources:
    archiving of, 119–20;
    budgeting for, 127–28;
    bundling of, 127–28;
    and confidentiality issues, 116–17;
    and copyright compliance, 117;
    and cost-reductions for libraries, 8;
    extent of, in libraries, 115–16;

health care institution administrators,
    expectations of, 8;
    integrity of, 116–17;
    Internet information concerning, 7;
    and librarian roles, 121–22;
    licensing of, 7, 27, 121–22;
    and print equivalents, 115–16;
    reserve collections, 117;
    and shelving space, effect on, 152;
    volatility of, 115
elevators, 165, 167
end-user searching, 108–9, 113–14
end-user training, 109, 113–14
Equal Employment Opportunity
    Commission, 45–46
Equal Pay Act, 1963, 60
ergonomics, 158–59, 167–68
evidence-based medicine, 4–5, 114
exhibits, 92–93, 163
exit interviews, 54

Fair Credit and Reporting Act, 1970,
    47–48
Fair Labor Standards Act, 1938, 60
federal libraries, 45, 63
fee-based services, 32–33
focus groups, 84
formula budgets, 22
The Foundation Center, 30
The Foundation Directory, 30
Friends of Libraries USA (FOLUSA), 32
friends of the library groups, 31–32, 91
fund raising:
    activities involved in, 29;
    for building, 138;
    funding proposal preparation, 30;
    and parent institution's policy, 28;
    planning for, 29;
    and site visits, 30–31;
    sources of funds, 30–33
funding proposals, preparation of, 30–31

Georgetown University Library
    Information System (LIS), 106
gophers, 111–12
GPEP Report. *See Physicians for the
    Twenty-First Century*
Grateful Med, 108
group study rooms, 156

health care institutions, 6, 24, 110. *See also*
    health care systems; hospitals
health care systems, 2–4, 9–10, 36
health information research:
    administration's role in, 189–91;
    behavioral studies in, 179–80;
    collaborative efforts in, 187–89;
    courses in, 174–75;
    evaluative: benchmark development,
        188; book availability studies, 182,
        184–86; comparisons in, 183;
        importance of, 175, 182;
        information retrieval studies, 182;
        lack of, 182; literature on, 182–83;
        need for, 189; output measures,
        182;
    and evidence-based librarianship, 174;
    flaws in, 183;
    importance of, 173–76, 182;
    institutional support for, 189–90;
    literature on, 174, 182–83;
    MLA role in, 173–74, 190–91;
    opportunities for, 189;
    patient outcome studies, 182;
    and practice guidelines, 174, 187;
    publication of results, 190.
    See also research
health professionals:
    document delivery for, 112–13, 180;
    education of, and technology, 109–10;
    and evidence-based practice, 4–5, 114;
    information needs of, 4–5, 9, 110–11;
    information-seeking behavior of, 4–5;
        78;
    and medical informatics, 110–11;
    online searching by, 108, 113–14;
    in primary care, 4;
    and problem-based learning, 5;
    and telehealth, 5;
    training support for, 4
health services research, 122
health sciences librarians:
    attributes of, 37–39;
    code of ethics for, 103;
    and collective bargaining, 46–47;
    consumer health information roles,
        3–4;
    core knowledge areas for, 38;
    and distance learning, 8, 118;

employer expectations for, 38;
    and electronic discussion lists, 112;
    and end-user training, 109, 113–14;
    in evidence-based practice projects, 5;
    flexibility in duties of, 42;
    and health information research, 174;
    and health services research, 122;
    and IAIMS, 6;
    job descriptions for, 39, 50;
    and job evaluation, 49;
    and knowledge management, 39, 122;
    life-long learning for, 103, 126;
    and marketing professionals, compared
        with, 75–76;
    and paraprofessionals, 42;
    performance standards for, 63 (*see also*
        performance evaluation; problem-
        based learning);
    professional development: activities
        involved in, 57; and continuing
        education, 12–14, 55–56; and job
        training, 56–57; and management
        training, 14; MLA role in, 12–13 (*see
        also Platform for Change*); new
        employee orientation in, 56; NLM
        role in, 13; plan for, 57–59;
        responsibility for, 12, 40, 54–55. *See
        also* staff development programs
    quality of work life, 66–68, 126;
    recruitment of, 13, 50–51 (*see also*
        recruitment, library);
    role of: as collaborator, 102; in
        consumer health services, 121; as
        educator, 109, 113–14; and research
        consultation, 9;
    and technology, 115, 120–23;
    skills: changes in, 36–37; and the
        current work force, 39;
        recommendations for, 13, 126,
        195–97; and technology, 125; value,
        by employers, 38;
    and technology training, 6–7, 125–26;
    and technostress, 126;
    titles for, 43, 125.
    See also hospital librarians
health sciences libraries:
    administration of. *See* health sciences
        library administration;
    antidiscrimination legislation in, 45;

buildings. *See* space planning, library;
competitive position of, 81;
corporate partners for, 32;
cost analysis in: automation effects,
    24–25; direct costs, 23; for fee-based
    services, 32–33; fixed costs, 24;
    importance of, 23–24; indirect costs,
    23–24; and leasing of services, 28;
    for serials, 26–27; variable costs, 24;
and cost increases of materials, 8, 25–26;
electronic collections in, 115–16 (*see
    also* electronic resources);
evidence-based librarianship in, 102–3,
    174;
friends groups for, 31, 91;
funding sources for, 29–32, 138 (*see
    also under* marketing);
and health care system changes, 9–10;
homepages for, 116;
and the IAIMS environment, 6, 80;
and information systems departments,
    5–6;
learning environment in, 126;
leasing services in, 28;
and managed care, 2;
marketing in. *See under* marketing;
off-site users, 116;
and the parent institution, 19, 102–3;
products, definition of, 80–81;
renovation of. *See* space planning,
    library;
research in administration's support
    for, 189–90; collaborative efforts in,
    187–89; examples of, 188. *See also*
    health information research
services in: definition of, 80–81; focus
    on, 102; space planning for. *See*
    space planning, library;
staff in: budgeting for, 128; and
    customer relations, 94;
    development of. *See* staff
    development programs; evaluation
    of. *See* performance evaluation;
    flexibility of duties, 42; fringe
    benefits for, 61; growth in size of,
    157–58; levels of, 41–2;
    management of (*see* health sciences
    library administration; human
    resources management); marketing

role, 76, 80, 89–90, 94; and minority
    recruitment, 46; new roles for, 42,
    158; and organizational structure,
    39–40; planning for, 41–42;
    recruitment of. *See* recruitment,
    library; salaries for, 59–60; space
    allocation for. *See under* space
    planning, library; teams, 43–45;
    technology training for, 125–26; and
    technostress, 126; titles for, 43. *See
    also* health sciences librarians;
    hospital librarians
stakeholders in, 79;
and stress, sources of, 67, 126;
technological development in. *See*
    technology, library;
and telehealth, 5;
types of, 41;
use by health professionals, 4, 78;
and user expectations, 7–9, 78, 142
health sciences library administration:
and change, importance of, 102–3;
educational preparation for, 13–14;
and ethics, importance of, 103;
and evidence-based librarianship,
    102–3;
financial management, 11; budgeting
    in, 8, 20–23, 127–28; cost
    determination, 23–28, 32–33; and
    licensing of electronic resources,
    27; and managed care, 19; and
    planning, 20;
and the health care environment, 101;
in health care systems, 9–10;
and leadership, 128–29;
and life-long learning, 103;
and marketing, 11–12;
and organizational structure, 10–11,
    125;
and the parent institution, 102–3;
principles of, 10;
and research, support for, 189–91;
risk-taking in, 14;
service evaluation in, 102;
skills needed for, 13, 195–97;
space planning for, 159;
staff involved in, 11;
technological challenges for, 11, 101–3,
    128–29;

and technology expertise, 11;
and time allocation, 12;
titles used in, 125
health sciences library consortia, 26–27
HealthWeb, 188
High Performance Computing and
    Communications Act, 118
hospital administrators, 8
hospital librarians:
    administrations' expectations of, 8;
    consumer health education role, 3–4;
    health professionals' expectations of, 9;
    and health services research, role in,
        121;
    information management role, 6;
    online training by, 109;
    responsibilities of, 41
hospital libraries:
    contracting for services in, 27–28;
    cost determination in, 24;
    and hospital mergers, 2–3;
    and JCAHO standards, 6, 8;
    journal usage study in, 188;
    marketing in, 83, 96;
    and outpatient service support, 3;
    staffing levels in, 41;
    value of, 37
hospitals:
    consumer health education in, 3–4;
    cost containment in, 2;
    decreased utilization of, 3;
    JCAHO requirements for, 6, 8;
    and managed care, 19;
    mergers between, 2–3
human resources management:
    affirmative action plans, 46, 51;
    antidiscrimination legislation, 45–46;
    collective bargaining, 46–47;
    compensation issues, 59–61;
    components of, 35–36, 40;
    of disabled workers, 48;
    employee safety, 47;
    evaluation of staff (*see* performance
        evaluation);
    flexibility of duties, 42;
    future issues in, for libraries, 68–69;
    job analysis, 48–50;
    job evaluation, 49;
    job titles, 43;

learning styles, 126;
legislation affecting, 45–48;
noncitizen hiring, 47;
objectives of, 40–41;
and the parent organization, 40, 48–50;
privacy of information, 47–48;
quality of work life, 66–68;
recruitment. *See* recruitment, library;
staff qualities needed in, 40;
staff training (*see* staff development
    programs);
staffing levels, 41–42;
of student workers, 43;
of teams, 43–45;
work schedules, 66
hypertext, 111–12

IAIMS, 6, 80, 110, 119
Immigration and Reform Control Act,
    1986, 47
information seeking behavior, 4, 5, 9, 78
information systems departments, 5–6
integrated library systems, 109
interlibrary lending, 105, 107–8, 112–13, 160
International Coalition of Library Consortia
    (ICOLC), 118–19
Internet:
    development of, 104–5;
    hospital administrators' expectations
        of, 8;
    licensing information from, 7;
    standards for data transmission over,
        104–5;
    and telecommunications costs for
        libraries, 24.
    See also World Wide Web
Internet Grateful Med, 113
intranets, 116

JCAHO, 6, 8
job analysis, 48–50
job descriptions, 39, 48–49
job evaluation, 49
job interviews, 52–53
JSTOR, 119–20

knowledge management, 11, 39, 122

leasing, 28

Library Administration and Management
    Association (LAMA), 137
library consortia, 115, 118–19
library development. *See* fund raising
*Library education and personnel
    utilization*, 43
licensing agreements, 7, 27, 121–22
line item budgets, 21–22
loading docks, 162
*Long-range Plan on the Education and
    Training of Health Sciences
    Librarians*, 40
lump sum budgets, 21

mailrooms, library, 162
managed care, 2, 4, 19
marketing:
    definition of, 77;
    in health sciences libraries: and
        advocacy, 79; the audit in, 82;
        budgeting for, 81–82; and
        competition review, 82–83;
        educational role of, 80, 93;
        environmental assessment in, 82;
        and innovation, 90; issues involved
        in, 76–77, 94–95; market analysis,
        82; market segmentation, 83;
        model, for strategies to use. *See*
        marketing mix; need for, 76, 78–80,
        97; to patients, 79; plan for, 79–81;
        and pricing, 87–88; and promotion.
        See promotional strategies; research
        techniques in, 82–84; scenarios for,
        95–96; staff involved in, 76, 80,
        89–90; and strategic planning,
        79–80; and strategies used, 90; and
        user needs, 75–76, 78, 84; and value
        of the library, 78–79;
    in hospital libraries, 83, 96;
    and marketing professionals, 75–76;
    in public libraries, 79;
    and selling, 75, 78;
    specialty areas in, 76 (*see also*
        advertising; marketing research
        techniques; promotional strategies);
    strategies used in, 77;
    and technology, 83;
    user surveys in, 78, 84
Marketing Is Everything, 76

marketing mix model, 84;
    and delivery of products and services,
        87;
    market share index, 86–87;
    political considerations, 89;
    portfolio mix model, 86–87;
    and pricing, 87–88;
    and product acceptance, 85;
    products and services life cycles,
        85–86;
    and promotion, 88–89
marketing research techniques, 83–84
Matheson report, 6, 36–37, 102
medical informatics:
    and AMIA, 118;
    challenges for, 119;
    definition of, 107;
    development of, 106–7;
    growth of, 110;
    in medical education, 109;
    in MLA, 111;
    NLM funding for, 110
Medical Library Association:
    and continuing education, 13;
    and librarian role definition, 37;
    Medical Informatics Section, 111;
    and professional development, 12–13,
        126, 195 (*see also Platform   for
        Change*)
    recruitment assistance from, 51;
    and research: bibliography on, 174,
        177; policy statement on, 173–74;
        recognition of importance of,
        190–91; Research Section, 191;
    Task Force on Knowledge and Skills,
        13
Medical School Objectives Project, 113
MEDLIB-L, 112
MEDLINE:
    CD-ROM access to, 108;
    development of, 105;
    end-user searching of, 108, 113–14;
    Web access to, 113–14
MELVYL System, 106
meta-analysis, 114, 122, 186–87

National Labor Relations Act, 1935, 46
National Laboratory for the Study of Rural
    Telemedicine, 5

National Library of Medicine:
 CD-ROM evaluation, 108;
 grants for libraries, 30;
 and IAIMS, 110;
 informatics funding, 110;
 librarian education and training grants,
  13, 40
Netwellness, 121

Occupational Safety and Health Act, 1970,
 47
OCLC, 105–6, 108, 119
Octanet, 107
OhioLINK, 115
OLDMEDLINE, 105
OPACs, 105–6, 108–9, 115;
Output Measures for Public Libraries, 183

packaging, promotional, 88–89
paraprofessionals:
 and levels of responsibility, 42, 49;
 and professional staff levels, 42;
 skills needed in, 39;
 titles for, 43
patient education, 79
penetration pricing, 88
performance budgets, 22
performance evaluation:
 in academic libraries, 64;
 and behavior, 62;
 criteria for, 63, 65;
 360-degree evaluation, 64;
 and disciplinary action, 66;
 and grievances, 65–66;
 interviews in, 65;
 and library goals, 62;
 peer review, 64;
 problems in, 61–62;
 for professional staff, 63;
 role of, 61;
 self-rating in, 64–65;
 of teams, 63–64;
 techniques used in, 62–63
Personnel Administration in Libraries, 47
PHILSOM, 105, 107
photocopiers, 164
Physicians for the Twenty-First Century, 109
Platform for Change, 12, 38–40, 50, 54–55,
 59, 195

primary care, 4
Privacy Act, 1974, 47–48
problem-based learning, 5, 8
professional development, librarian,
 12–14, 40, 54–56. *See also* staff
 development programs program
 budgets, 22
promotional strategies:
 advertising, 88;
 advisory group role in, 91;
 consumer information services as, 79,
  94;
 customer services, staff training in, 94;
 definition of, 88;
 direct mailings, 90;
 exhibits as, 92–93;
 friends of the library groups, 91;
 help desks as, 93;
 library cooperative efforts in, 90;
 mass media in, 92;
 multimedia as, 92;
 packaging as, 88–89;
 public relations as, 89;
 publications as, 91–92;
 telephone solicitation, 90;
 training sessions as, 93
public libraries, 79, 182
public relations, 89
public services, 160, 163–64
PubMed, 113
PubMed Central, 120

quality of work life, 66–68
QuickDoc, 108

rare books, 154
receiving areas, library, 162
recruitment, library:
 and affirmative action, 46, 51;
 competition in, 51;
 and cover letters, 52;
 of disabled workers, 48;
 electronic job listings for, 51;
 and exit interviews, 54;
 and expectations of employers, 38–39;
 job interviews, 52–53;
 job offers, 53;
 and knowledge management, 39;
 MLA role in, 51;

of noncitizens, 47;
plans for, 50–51;
reference checks, 52;
and retention, 54;
resumes, 52;
search committee role, 51–52;
strategies used in, 50
reference desks, 164
reference stacks, 153–54
research:
    application of findings of, 185–86;
    assumptions in, 180–81;
    bias in, 178, 181;
    critical incident technique in, 178;
    data collection in, 187–89;
    descriptive statistics in, 176;
    dissemination of results of, 180,
        183–84, 190;
    evaluative, 175–76, 181–83;
    field testing in, 186;
    fraud in, 183–84;
    hypothesis testing in, 178, 180–81;
    inferential statistics in, 176;
    objectives of, 175, 179;
    prediction in, 177;
    probability in, 176–77;
    qualitative, 178, 181, 185;
    quantitative, 176–78, 181, 183;
    reliability of findings, 179–81;
    and replication, 185–85;
    sampling in, 177;
    significance in, 177;
    steps in, 175–76;
    survey, 177;
    theoretical models, 178, 180–81;
    validity in, 179–81;
    variables in, 176, 184–86.
    See also health information research
Research Libraries Group, 106, 112
research, library, 78
research, medical, 9
responsibility-centered management,
    22–23

salaries, librarian, 59–60
search committees, 51–52
seating, library, 155–57, 168;
security, library, 167–68
serials, 25–27, 154;

shelving, library, 151–54, 167;
site visits, 30–31
skimming price strategy, 88
space planning, library:
    and access *versus* ownership, 135;
    architects: communication with,
        146–47; fee negotiation with, 145; in
        the planning team, 140–41;
        selection of, 143–45;
    and bidding for construction, 149;
    budgeting for, 137–38;
    building effectiveness and efficiency,
        150;
    building program plans: architect role
        in, 146–47; consultants used for,
        136; definition of, 136; elements in,
        136–37, 146; importance of, 136;
        literature on, 137, 199–203; staff
        involvement in, 136; timing of,
        135–36; verification of, 146–47;
        writing of, 136–37;
    charette technique in, 146–47;
    for circulation desks, 163–64;
    for collections, 151–54;
    for conservation activities, 163;
    construction documents, 148–49;
    and dedication of buildings, 169–70;
    design development phase in, 148;
    and effectiveness of building, 150;
    and efficiency of building, 150;
    elevators, 165, 167;
    environmental considerations, 166–67;
    ergonomic considerations, 158–59,
        167–68;
    for exhibit preparations, 163;
    funding sources for, 138;
    interior design, 168–69;
    lighting considerations, 167;
    literature on, 137, 199–203;
    lobby space, 163;
    and mission of the library, 134;
    and move into new space, 169;
    and the parent organization, 134;
    planning team: importance of, 139–40;
        literature on, 140; members of,
        140–42; and project manager's role,
        140;
    preparation for, 135;
    for print collections, 135;

for public amenities, 164–65;
for receiving areas, 162;
safety issues, 167–68;
schematic design phase, 147–48, 157;
for seating space, public, 155–57, 168;
and shape of building, 151;
and site for building, 138–39, 151;
and size of building, 151;
staff roles in: architect selection,
    143–45; construction document
    review, 148–49; design phases,
    147–48; final construction phase,
    169; importance of, 136, 140;
    project management, 140, 143, 145,
    149; for public services space
    determination, 160;
staff space: for access services, 159; for
    administration, 159; calculation of,
    157–58; for conferences, 161;
    ergonomic aspects, 158–59, 167;
    and functional relationships, 157;
    future projections for, 158; for
    interlibrary loan services, 160; for
    lounge, 162; planning for, 157; for
    public services, 160, 163–64; for
    storage, 162; for systems
    department, 161; for teaching, 157,
    167–68; for technical services,
    160–61; technology requirements.
    See under technology, library;
    for stairs, 167;
wallboarding technique in, 146–47
Special Libraries Association, 13, 196–97
staff development programs:
    assessment of, 58;
    benefits of, 55;
    and continuing education, 55–56;
    in customer relations, 94;
    development activities in, 57;
    goals of, 57;
    and individual plans, 55;
    job training in, 56–57;
    library responsibility for, 54–55;
    and needs identification, 57–58;
    orientation for new employees in, 56;
    plans for, 57–59;
    systematic approach to, 55;
    in technology, 125–26;
    training resources for, 58

Stress and Burnout in Library Service, 67
student workers, 43
support staff. *See* paraprofessionals
survey methodologies, 188–89;
systems department, library, 161

tables, library, 156
Taft-Hartley Act, 1946, 46
teams, 43–45, 63–64
technical services department, 160–61
technology, library:
    archiving of electronic documents,
        119–20;
    authentication issues, 116–17;
    budgeting for, 8, 127–28;
    and capital expenses, 25;
    CD-ROM, 108;
    collaborative projects in, 115,
        118–120;
    confidentiality issues, 116–17;
    cost determination for, 24–25;
    database proliferation, 113;
    distance learning, 117;
    for document delivery, 112–13;
    electronic communication methods,
        112;
    electronic reserves, 117;
    equipment life cycles, 127;
    evidence-based medicine
        requirements, 114;
    and the health care environment, 101;
    homepages, 116;
    hypertext, 111–12;
    for ILL activities, 105, 107–8, 112–13;
    and information management, 6;
    and the information systems
        department, 5–6;
    integrated library systems, 109;
    and integrity of information, 116–17;
    intranets, 116;
    and leadership requirements, 128–29;
    licensing issues, 7, 27, 121–22;
    and marketing, 80;
    in medical education, 109–10;
    online database searching, 6, 105,
        108–9, 113–14;
    OPAC development, 105–6, 108–9, 115;
    and organizational structure, 124–25;
    and paradigm shift, 103–5;

and the parent organization, 102–3;
and performance measures, 124;
research needed in, 189;
reviews of, 104;
and role of libraries, 101, 120–23;
and role of library staff, 6, 11, 36, 68–69, 120–23;
for serials tracking, 105;
staff involved with, 11, 68–69;
and staff training, 6–7, 125–26;
space planning for: cabling, 166; electricity, 166; environmental concerns, 166–67; ergonomic concerns, 158–59, 167; and flexibility, 134–35, 142, 165–66; importance of, 166; lighting, 167; microcomputer classrooms, 157; public workstations, 156, 166–67; questions to consider, 150–51, 166; seating requirements, 155; staff involved in, 142, 150;
survey of, 111;
and systems integration, 110–11;

and transitional needs, 6;
and user expectations, 7–9, 123–24;
and value of the library, 101–2, 120;
and volatility of resources, 115
telefacsimile, 108
telehealth, 5
telemedicine, 118

Unified Medical Language System, 111
user groups, computer, 91
user surveys, 78, 84
Value of the Hospital Library, 37

Western Governors University (WGU), 117, 122–23
workstations, public, 157, 166–67
World Wide Web:
development of, 111;
homepages for libraries, 116;
MEDLINE access on, 113–14.
See also Internet

zero-based budgets, 22

Author Biographies

Joan S. Ash holds joint appointments in the library and in the Division of Medical Informatics and Outcomes Research, School of Medicine, at Oregon Health Sciences University. She had been a reference librarian, library administrator, and IAIMS coordinator at various times in her career prior to joining the core informatics teaching faculty full-time. In addition to her library degree, she has an MBA with a marketing major and a Ph.D. in systems science–business administration. She has been active in MLA and AMIA (the American Medical Informatics Association), having served on the board of directors and editorial boards for both organizations.

Prudence W. Dalrymple was appointed dean of the Graduate School of Library and Information Science at Dominican University in River Forest, Illinois, in 1997. Previously she directed the Office for Accreditation at the American Library Association and was on the faculty at the University of Illinois. She has worked as an academic health sciences librarian and a hospital librarian as well as an educator and administrator. She has been a member of the Medical Library Association since 1978 and is a distinguished member of the Academy of Health Information Professionals. She chaired the task force that created the MLA research policy "Using Scientific Evidence to Improve Health Information Practice" and currently serves on the National Library of Medicine's Biomedical Library Review Committee. She has taught health sciences librarianship and has published widely on topics relevant to health sciences and to research and evaluation.

Ellen G. Detlefsen is a tenured faculty member in the School of Information Sciences at the University of Pittsburgh, with joint appointments in the Women's Studies Program and the Center for Biomedical Informatics. She directs the university's program in medical librarianship. She was educated at Smith College and holds her M.S. and doctorate from the Columbia University School of Library Service. Her areas of expertise and teaching are biomedical and health sciences information, medical informatics, and resources and services for special populations such as patients, health care consumers, and the aging and their caregivers. She is an active member of MLA, in which she is chair of the Medical Library Education Section; she also currently serves on Chapter Council of MLA and on the national MLANET Editorial Board. She is currently project director for the Highmark Minority Health Link initiative, which seeks to build minority-sensitive consumer health materials for the African-American communities of western Pennsylvania.

Barbara A. Epstein is associate director for administrative services at the University of Pittsburgh Health Sciences Library System and a core faculty member of the university's Center for Biomedical Informatics. Formerly, she was director of the library of the Western Psychiatric Institute and Clinic. She has been actively involved in the Medical Library Association and other professional associations, having served as officer in several sections, chapters, and committees and president of the Association of Mental Health Librarians. Her professional interests include planning and management of library services in academic health centers, development of outreach programs, and education and training of health sciences librarians. She is a distinguished member of the Academy of Health Information Professionals.

Rick B. Forsman directs the Denison Memorial Library at the University of Colorado Health Sciences Center in Denver. He has chaired and served on more than a dozen committees, sections, and task forces of the Medical Library Association and was named a fellow of MLA in 1999. In addition, he has served on the Association of Academic Health Sciences Libraries' board of directors, the American Library Association's Committee on Accreditation, and the International Federation of Library Associations' Biological and Medical Sciences Libraries Section. He remains avidly interested in technological projects and advises on campus and university-wide information competencies and technology policy. A frequent scuba diver and international traveler, Forsman is seeking venture capital to develop UNIP, the world's first Underwater Network for Information Professionals.

Carol Jenkins has been director of the Health Sciences Library, University of North Carolina at Chapel Hill since 1986, and she held prior administrative positions at the University of Maryland, University of Virginia, and Oregon Health Sciences University. She received funded management traineeships at the University of Cincinnati and the Summer Institute for Women in Higher Education Administration at Bryn Mawr College. She has been active on campuses in many areas including women's concerns, planning and budgeting, copyright, and library issues. She has published and presented papers in the areas of information outreach services and educational preparation of health sciences librarians for future roles, some grant supported. She has served as president of the Association of Academic Health Sciences Libraries and is active in MLA at the chapter and national levels. She served on the

MLA board of directors and will serve as MLA president in 2002. The Mid-Atlantic Chapter, MLA, chose her as Librarian of the Year, in 1999.

Patricia C. Mickelson has more than twenty-six years of experience in supervision and administration in large academic health sciences libraries. She is director of the Health Sciences Library System at the University of Pittsburgh. Previous positions include serving as deputy director of the Health Sciences Library at the University of Maryland and head of public services at the Welch Medical Library, Johns Hopkins University. In 1999 she served as president of the Association of Academic Health Sciences Libraries. Her professional interests include leadership development, effecting the transition to the digital library, and the integration of information in the academic health center.

Lynn Kasner Morgan is assistant dean for Information Resources and Systems, research associate professor of medical education, and director of the Gustave L. and Janet W. Levy Library at the Mount Sinai School of Medicine. She has over twenty years of experience in administering library and computing services. For seven years she taught biomedical communication for the Columbia University School of Library Service; for six years she taught health sciences librarianship for the Queens College School of Library and Information Studies. In addition to serving on numerous MLA committees, she has been president of the Association of Academic Health Science Library Directors and a member of the board of trustees of the Medical Library Center of New York and the New York Metropolitan Reference and Resources Library Council.

Audrey Powderly Newcomer is the director of the Health Sciences Center Library at Saint Louis University in St. Louis, Missouri. During the 1998-99 academic year, she served as interim associate vice president for information technology services for the university. She has been active in technical services and library automation since the beginning of her career in 1976. Previous to her position at Saint Louis University, she was director of the Library at University of Arkansas for Medical Sciences. Active in the Medical Library Association, she has served on the board of directors and chaired Section Council. She is the 1988 recipient of the Estelle Brodman Award for the Academic Medical Librarian of the Year. She currently serves on the board of directors for the Association of Academic Health Sciences Libraries.

Mary Joan (M.J.) Tooey is the deputy director of the Health Sciences and Human Services Library at the University of Maryland where she has worked, in various capacities, for fourteen years. One of the positions she held there was that of project manager for the new library, which opened in 1998, where she was involved with every aspect of the building, from the selection of the architects to the actual construction and opening of the building. She is a member of the board of directors of the Medical Library Association where she is chair of Chapter Council. In 1997 she received the MLA Estelle Brodman Award for Academic Medical Librarian of the Year, and she is a distinguished member of the Academy of Health Information Professionals. She has also served as the chair of the Public Services Section of MLA and chair of the Mid-Atlantic Chapter. She has over fifty publication and presentations in diverse areas such as technology, education, service, and informatics.

Frieda O. Weise is executive director of the Health Sciences and Human Services Library at the University of Maryland, Baltimore Campus. She has been a medical librarian for more than twenty-five years and has gained broad experience and knowledge in library administration, information technology, and library buildings. Her professional contributions include teaching for MLA, publications, presentations, and MLA activities. She has coauthored several papers and a symposium on building the library of the future. She served as the eightieth president of the Medical Library Association in 2000.

Elizabeth H. Wood was most recently head of research and reference services at Oregon Health Sciences University. She has served MLA as member and chair of the Books Panel, a member of the editorial board of the *Bulletin,* chair of the Public Services and Pharmacy & Drug Information Sections, a member of Section Council, and a member of numerous other section and chapter committees. She is author of a chapter in the educational services volume in this series. Ms. Wood has been chapter member of the year for ASIS and is also a member of AMIA and a distinguished member of the Academy of Health Information Professionals.